Bitter Legacy

Christopher Lee Roeters

Published by Christopher Lee Roeters, 2026.

BITTER LEGACY

First edition. February 23, 2026.

ISBN: 979-8233832314

Written by Christopher Lee Roeters.

Table of Contents

Prologue

Bitter Legacy

The story of the PBB poisoning in Michigan is not just a historical event; it is a living, breathing legacy that continues to shape the lives of those who were affected. Unlike the movie 'Bitter Harvest', which focused on the immediate aftermath of the 1973 cattle feed contamination, 'Bitter Legacy' is a deeply personal account of what it means to survive—not just the initial crisis, but the lifelong consequences that followed. This is not a story about triumph over adversity; it is a story about enduring, adapting, and finding meaning in a life forever altered by a preventable tragedy.

My name is Christopher Lee Roeters, and I am one of the prenatal victims of the PBB poisoning. My story begins before I was even born, in the womb of my mother, who unknowingly consumed contaminated dairy products during her pregnancy. Like thousands of others in Michigan, she had no idea that the milk she drank, the butter she spread on her toast, and the cheese she enjoyed were laced with polybrominated biphenyls—a toxic chemical mistakenly mixed into cattle feed. By the time the error was discovered, it was too late. The poison had already entered the food chain, affecting not only the cattle but also the people who consumed their products.

The immediate effects of the poisoning were devastating. Thousands of cattle died, their bodies riddled with tumors and lesions. Tens of thousands of bald eagles, consuming water that had contact with the ground water of which the buried cattle affected, also perished. But the human toll was far more insidious. Unborn children, like me, were exposed to PBBs during critical stages of development. Many did not survive. Those of us who did were left with a legacy of health problems that would haunt us for the rest of our lives.

My earliest memories are not of playgrounds or birthday parties, but of doctor's offices and hospital rooms. As a child, I was plagued by a host of medical issues that no one could fully explain. I suffered from chronic fatigue, frequent infections, and developmental delays. My immune system seemed to be perpetually on the verge of collapse, and my parents were told that I would likely never lead a "normal" life.

Doctors were baffled by my condition. At the time, the long-term effects of prenatal PBB exposure were not well understood. It wasn't until years later, when researchers began to connect the dots between the poisoning and the health problems of those exposed, that my symptoms started to make sense. By then, the damage had already been done.

Growing up, I was acutely aware that I was different from other children. While my peers were running and playing, I was often too weak to join them. I missed countless days of school due to illness, and I struggled to keep up with my classmates academically. The physical toll of my condition was compounded by the emotional burden of feeling like an outsider. I didn't understand why I was so sick, and neither did anyone else.

As I grew older, I became determined to understand the root cause of my health problems. With a little research I found out about the PBB poisoning, but it wasn't until I began researching the incident myself that I fully grasped its magnitude. I learned about the chemical plant where the mistake had occurred, the identical bags of feed supplement and fire retardant that had been stacked side by side, and the catastrophic chain of events that followed.

I also learned about the failures of the system that allowed the contamination to go unnoticed for so long. State authorities, fearing panic, delayed going public with the facts. As a result, people continued to consume contaminated dairy products for months, even after the problem had been identified. The consequences of this delay were far-reaching and, in many cases, irreversible.

Reading about the incident was both enlightening and infuriating. On one hand, it gave me a sense of validation. For the first time, I had a plausible explanation for my health problems. On the other hand, it filled me with anger. How could such a mistake have happened? Why weren't more precautions in place to prevent it? And why had it taken so long for the truth to come to light?

The PBB poisoning was a wake-up call for many industries, leading to significant changes in how chemicals are handled, labeled, and tested. Bar coding and different packaging have made mix-ups far less likely, and advances in technology have improved our ability to detect harmful substances in food and the environment. Animal welfare practices have also evolved, with more humane methods of euthanasia now standard.

But while these changes are important, they do little to ease the burden of those who were already affected. For people like me, the legacy of the poisoning is not just a historical footnote; it is a daily reality. The health problems I face are a constant reminder of the mistakes of the past, and the lessons learned have come at a great cost.

This is not a story about overcoming adversity. It is a story about surviving—about learning to live with the hand you've been dealt, even when the odds are stacked against you. My life has been shaped by the PBB poisoning in ways that I am still discovering. Some days, the weight of it feels unbearable. Other days, I find strength in the knowledge that I am not alone.

There are thousands of others like me—people who were exposed to PBBs prenatally or in early childhood, and who continue to grapple with the consequences. We are a community bound by a shared experience, united by a legacy that none of us chose but all of us must bear.

The story of the PBB poisoning is not just a cautionary tale; it is a call to action. It is a reminder that the choices we make—or fail to make—can have far-reaching consequences. It is a plea for greater transparency, accountability, and compassion in the face of crisis. And it is a testament to the resilience of the human spirit, even in the face of unimaginable challenges.

As I write this, I am acutely aware that my story is just one of many. There are countless others who have been affected by the PBB poisoning, each with their own unique experiences and perspectives. My hope is that by sharing my story, I can shed light on the ongoing impact of this tragedy and inspire others to take action to prevent similar incidents in the future.

The legacy of the PBB poisoning is a bitter one, but it is also a powerful reminder of the importance of vigilance, accountability, and compassion. It is a legacy that I will carry with me for the rest of my life, and one that I hope will serve as a lesson for generations to come.

This is not just my story. It is our story. And it is far from over.

—

As I reflect on my life and the challenges I have faced, I am reminded of the strength and resilience that have carried me through. The legacy of the PBB poisoning is a heavy one, but it is also a testament to the power of the human spirit. Despite the obstacles, I have found ways to adapt, to persevere, and to find meaning in my experiences.

My hope is that 'Bitter Legacy' will serve as a reminder of the importance of learning from the past, and of the need to continue fighting for a safer, more just world. The lessons of the PBB poisoning are not just about preventing future tragedies; they are about honoring the lives of those who were affected, and ensuring that their stories are never forgotten.

This is my legacy. This is our legacy. And it is one that I will continue to carry with pride.

—

The Bald Eagles: A Parallel Tragedy

The PBB poisoning did not only affect humans and livestock; it also had a devastating impact on wildlife, particularly the bald eagle population. Once treated as vermin and hunted to near extinction, bald eagles faced a new threat in the mid-20th century: human-made chemicals like DDT and PCBs.

The Michigan Bald Eagle Biomonitoring Project, a 57-year effort to track toxic chemical levels in eagles, revealed the extent of the damage. Eagles near the Great Lakes had toxicity levels six times higher than those in other regions, leading to lower birth rates and a host of health problems. The project's early research played a crucial role in raising awareness about the dangers of these chemicals and contributed to the eventual bans on DDT and PCBs in the 1970s.

Michigan's eagle population, which had dwindled to just 52 breeding pairs by 1961, began to recover following the bans and the establishment of protected habitats like the Detroit River International Wildlife Refuge. By 2019, the state was home to an estimated 900 breeding pairs—a testament to the resilience of nature when given a chance to heal.

The story of the bald eagles serves as a poignant parallel to the human experience of the PBB poisoning. Both are stories of survival, resilience, and the enduring impact of human actions on the environment. And both serve as a reminder of the importance of vigilance, accountability, and compassion in the face of crisis.

This is not just my story. It is our story. And it is far from over.

Chapter 1

I was born on May 24, 1973, in Traverse City, Michigan, at the Osteopathic hospital. My arrival into the world was marked by neither fanfare nor celebration, but rather by the quiet chaos of a family already unraveling. My biological mother, Sandy Williams, and my biological father, Lionel Lee Cryderman, were young and ill-prepared for the challenges of parenthood. They lived in Mancelona, a small town in northern Michigan, where the rolling hills and dense forests masked the turmoil within their home.

I was the first of three children they would have together, and from the very beginning, my life was shaped by instability. My mother struggled with personal issues that spilled over into her marriage, creating a volatile environment. Arguments were frequent, and the tension between my parents was palpable. Child Protective Services became a recurring presence in our lives, intervening multiple times to remove me and my younger siblings from the home. By the time I was three and a half years old, I had already experienced more upheaval than most children do in a lifetime.

In early 1977, I was placed in yet another foster home. This time, however, it would be different. This time, it would become permanent. Mary and Berend Roeters of Charlevoix, Michigan, opened their home to me, and though the formal adoption wouldn't take place until I was around nine years old, they became my family from the moment I stepped through their door.

The Roeters household was a bustling one. At the time I arrived, they were already fostering two other children: Earlene Jackson and Brian Brickner. Their only biological child, Berend Jr., was also part of the mix. As the youngest at just three and a half years old, I was the new addition to a family that was still figuring itself out.

Mary and Berend were kind-hearted people who believed in providing a safe and nurturing environment for children in need. They took their role as foster parents seriously, offering stability and love to those who had known little of either. But fitting into this new family wasn't easy for me. The scars of my early years ran deep, and I carried with me the weight of neglect and abuse that had marked my first few years of life.

From an early age, it was clear that I was different. I struggled with learning and developmental issues that set me apart from other children my age. My speech was garbled and difficult to understand, a result of both hearing problems and the trauma I had endured. By the time I was four, hearing aids were installed, which helped improve my speech over time. But the damage had already been done. I was approximately two years behind my peers academically and socially, a gap that would take years to close.

My health was another constant source of concern. I suffered from chronic stomach issues that left me feeling nauseous and weak much of the time. These symptoms were dismissed as childhood ailments, but in hindsight, they were likely early signs of the PBB poisoning that had affected me prenatally. Unfortunately, this connection wouldn't be made until decades later, leaving my adoptive parents in the dark about the true cause of my struggles.

Perhaps the most striking evidence of my troubled early years was the way I communicated. My adoptive mother, Mary, often recalled that when I first arrived in their home, it was as if I spoke my own language. I used repetitive words to describe specific objects or actions, a coping mechanism born out of neglect and abuse. It took time and patience for me to unlearn these habits and adapt to the world around me.

Adjusting to life with the Roeters family was a slow and often painful process. While Mary and Berend did their best to provide a loving and stable environment, I struggled to feel like I belonged. My relationship with Brian, one of the other foster children, was particularly fraught. He was older and more assertive, and our interactions were often marked by conflict. But the problems with Brian went far beyond typical sibling rivalry.

What I didn't understand at the time, and what my adoptive parents were unaware of, was that Brian was sexually abusing both me and Berend Jr., the Roeters' natural child. This abuse added another layer of trauma to an already fractured childhood. It was a secret I carried for years, too young to fully comprehend what was happening and too afraid to speak up. The shame and confusion I felt during that time only deepened my sense of isolation and made it even harder to trust those around me.

Some of the conflicts between Brian and me stemmed from my health issues, which neither of us fully understood at the time. But the abuse was a shadow that loomed over everything, a hidden wound that would take years to heal. It wasn't until much later in life that I began to process what had happened and understand the profound impact it had on me.

The Roeters family's frequent moves added another layer of complexity to my childhood. Berend's job working for area hospitals took us from Michigan to Colorado, then to Alaska, and eventually back to Michigan. These moves disrupted any sense of continuity I might have had, making it difficult to form lasting friendships or feel rooted in one place. They also kept my adoptive parents from uncovering the truth about my prenatal exposure to

PBB. By the time we returned to Michigan, I was an adult, and the damage had long since been done.

Looking back, it's clear that my early years were shaped by forces beyond my control. The neglect and abuse I experienced before entering the foster system left lasting scars, both physical and emotional. The PBB poisoning, though unknown to me at the time, added another layer of complexity to my struggles. It wasn't until much later in life that I would begin to piece together the full picture of how these factors had shaped me.

But even in the midst of these challenges, there were glimmers of hope. The Roeters family, despite their limitations, gave me a chance at a better life. They provided the stability and love I so desperately needed, even if they couldn't fully understand the depth of my struggles. And though my journey has been far from easy, it is a testament to the resilience of the human spirit—a resilience that would carry me through the years to come.

This is where my story begins: not with a clean slate, but with a fractured past and an uncertain future. It is a story of survival, of finding light in the darkest of places, and of learning to navigate a world that often feels stacked against you.

—

Many of the healtin problems I dealt with as a young child would have been much better understood by my adoptive parents if they had known about the PBB poisoning I had been exposed to prenatally. But because I was taken away from my biological family at such a young age, and because my adoptive parents moved frequently—first within Michigan and later, when I was 10 years old, to Colorado—there was no way for them to connect my symptoms to the poisoning. The effects of PBB on survivors weren't thoroughly investigated until a few years after I was born, and by then, I was just one of many children scattered across the country, adopted into different families and relocated far from the epicenter of the crisis.

The companies and agencies responsible for investigating the poisoning had no way of tracking me or my younger biological siblings, who had also been adopted into separate homes. As a result, my adoptive parents were left in the dark, grappling with a series of mysterious health issues that no one could fully explain.

Most of my symptoms seemed, at first glance, like common childhood ailments. I suffered from chronic stomach issues, which were often dismissed as typical upset stomachs. My hearing problems were obvious from the start, and the resulting speech impediment was one of the first clues that something was wrong. But the most striking and visible sign that something was amiss was my complete inability to grow hair. From the day I was born to this very day, I have never been able to grow a single hair anywhere on my body. This unusual condition became the focus of countless medical tests and appointments, as my adoptive parents sought answers to a question no one could answer.

By the time we moved to Colorado, there was still no widespread national news about the PBB poisoning in northern Michigan. My parents had no clue about the poisoning, and neither did the doctors who ran test after test, trying to figure out why I couldn't grow hair. No one connected the dots between my stomach issues, hearing loss, inability to grow hair, and other problems like my brittle bones. I can't count how many times I accidentally broke a tooth, separated a rib, or fractured other bones under circumstances that would have been harmless for any other child.

While many of my symptoms were likely linked to PBB exposure, some were unrelated but equally misunderstood. For example, I was lactose intolerant, a condition my adoptive parents were unfamiliar with. They had fostered other children and, by the time we moved to Colorado, had two more natural children of their own—Meaghan and Pieter—but none of them had experienced lactose intolerance. It's possible that the PBB poisoning exacerbated this condition, though I've never found any research to confirm a direct link.

Another obvious issue was my inability to gain much body weight. No matter how much I ate, I remained thin and frail, a fact that worried my parents and baffled doctors. Combined with my other symptoms, it painted a picture of a child whose body was fundamentally different, though no one could say why.

My adoptive parents did everything they could to help me. They pushed for tests, sought out specialists, and never stopped looking for answers. But without knowledge of the PBB poisoning, they were fighting a battle without all the necessary information. The doctors we saw were equally perplexed, focusing on individual symptoms rather than seeing the bigger picture.

It wassn't until much later in life, when I began researching the PBB crisis and its long-term effects, that I started to understand the root causes of my health issues. By then, the damage had been done, and I had spent decades grappling with the physical and emotional toll of a condition no one had diagnosed.

Looking back, it's clear that my early years were shaped by forces beyond my control. The PBB poisoning, combined with the neglect and abuse I experienced before entering the foster system, left me with a legacy of health problems that would affect me for the rest of my life. But it also taught me resilience—the ability to adapt, to endure, and to keep moving forward even when the odds are stacked against you.

—-

Growing up, I had friends like most typical children. For the most part, I participated in outside activities, including sleepovers at friends' homes and having friends stay over at mine. These experiences were a normal part of childhood, but they were often overshadowed by the constant discomfort of my upset stomach and the emotional toll of being different.

My inability to grow hair and my hearing issues made me a target for teasing from other children. Even with hearing aids, which were much larger and more noticeable back then compared to today's discreet designs, I still struggled to hear perfectly. The hearing aids themselves became a source of ridicule, and I often chose to go without them to avoid the teasing. This meant that much of my childhood was spent navigating social situations with limited hearing, a fact that many of my peers didn't realize. The combination of my baldness and hearing challenges made me stand out in ways I couldn't control, and the constant teasing took a toll on my self-esteem.

By the time I was old enough to start elementary school in Michigan, it was clear that I wasn't ready for kindergarten, despite being the right age. My developmental delays, a result of both my early trauma and the lingering effects of PBB exposure, put me behind my peers academically. A year later, I was finally enrolled in kindergarten in Boyne City, Michigan. But even after completing kindergarten, I wasn't ready for first grade. Instead, I was placed in a program called Junior Primary, a half-step between kindergarten and first grade designed to help children who needed extra time to catch up.

This pattern continued throughout my early education. By the time I was 10 years old and my family moved to Colorado, I was only in the third grade—two years behind most of my peers. Being older than the other children in my grade added another layer of difficulty to my social interactions. I was always the "big kid" in class, a fact that made me feel even more out of place.

Despite these challenges, I was outgoing with my immediate friends. However, when it came to meeting new people, I was painfully shy. This shyness stayed with me for most of my life, and I typically kept only a handful of close friends at any given time. Friends came and went, as they do for most people, but the ones who stayed became an important part of my support system.

Moving to Colorado at the age of 10 marked a turning point in my life. My adoptive father, Berend Sr., got me involved in Cub Scouts, and it was one of the best things that could have happened to me. Cub Scouts opened the door to new friendships and experiences. For the first time, I was part of a group where respect was a core value, and the teasing I had endured for so long was almost nonexistent. The other children in the Scouts accepted me for who I was, and I finally felt like I belonged somewhere.

When I turned 13, still living in Craig, Colorado, I became eligible for another program that I had been eagerly looking forward to: the Police Explorers. This program, run by the local police department, allowed teenagers to ride along with officers and observe their daily routines. It was an incredible opportunity to learn about law enforcement and contribute to the community in a meaningful way.

As a Police Explorer, I was paired with an officer and spent time in a patrol car, observing everything from routine traffic stops to community outreach efforts. While we were never placed in dangerous situations, the experience gave me a sense of purpose and responsibility. Like Cub Scouts, the Police Explorers program was another environment where I felt accepted and valued. The other participants and the officers I worked with treated me with respect, and I was able to make new friends without the fear of being teased or judged.

These programs—Cub Scouts and the Police Explorers—played a crucial role in helping me find my place in the world. They provided a sense of structure and belonging that I had been missing for much of my childhood. For the first time, I felt like I was part of something bigger than myself, and that feeling made all the difference.

Looking back, I can see how these experiences shaped me. They taught me the value of community, the importance of respect, and the power of perseverance. They also showed me that, despite the challenges I faced, there were places where I could thrive and people who would accept me for who I was.

—-

Cub Scouts had been a safe haven for me, a place where I felt accepted and valued. But as I grew older, the natural progression was to transition into Boy Scouts. While this was meant to be an advancement—a kind of graduation—it felt like a daunting change to me. I've never been comfortable with change, a trait that has stayed with me to some extent even today. The new structure, new expectations, and new dynamics of Boy Scouts made me uneasy, and shortly after joining, I made the difficult decision to step away from the program altogether.

This pattern of struggling with change and unfamiliar situations extended beyond Boy Scouts. Throughout my childhood, I often reacted to circumstances differently than most other children. Looking back, I think a large part of this was due to an underlying lack of trust and a constant, low-level anxiety that colored my interactions with the world. This anxiety affected not only my experience with Boy Scouts but also my time in the Police Explorers program.

The Police Explorers program had been a bright spot in my life, giving me a sense of purpose and belonging. But as I grew more comfortable with the officers I worked with, I began to see them as peers rather than authority figures. This was a mistake on my part. One day, in a moment of excitement and friendliness, I gave a female police officer a friendly pat on the back. It was an innocent gesture, born of the kind of enthusiasm that children naturally have, but it was misinterpreted as something more serious. As a result, I was removed from the program.

The loss of the Police Explorers was a blow. It wasn't just the end of an activity I enjoyed; it felt like the loss of a community where I had finally started to feel like I belonged. The experience left me feeling misunderstood and isolated, reinforcing the anxiety and mistrust that had always been a part of my life.

Around this time, my oldest foster sister, Earlene, moved to Craig, Colorado, with her two children, Warren and Joshua. Earlene had initially stayed in Michigan, living on a reservation in the Upper Peninsula where she was native to. But she felt the need to be closer to our family, and her move to Craig brought her back into my life in a meaningful way.

Earlene and I had always been close, and her presence in Craig was a source of comfort for me. Shortly after she arrived, I moved into an apartment with her and her children. This change was both exciting and unsettling. On one hand, I was thrilled to be living with Earlene, who felt like a true sibling to me. On the other hand, the move disrupted the living structure that had been so important to me. Stability and routine were everything to me, and this sudden shift was a shock to my system.

The arrangement was temporary, lasting only until I finished the school year. After that, I would relocate to Golden, Colorado, where my adoptive father, Berend Sr., had taken a new job. While I was excited to be with my parents again, the move to Golden came with a significant downside: it meant leaving behind the handful of close friends I had made in Craig.

Moving to Golden was a mixed experience. On one hand, it was good to be back with my parents and younger siblings, Meaghan and Pieter and older brother Berend Jr. On the other hand, the move severed the connections I had worked so hard to build in Craig. Making new friends had never been easy for me, and the thought of starting over in a new place was daunting.

The loss of my friends in Craig was a reminder of how much I valued the few close relationships I had. Those friendships had been a lifeline for me, providing a sense of belonging and acceptance that I struggled to find elsewhere. Starting over in Golden meant rebuilding that sense of connection from scratch, a challenge that felt overwhelming at the time.

Looking back, I can see how these experiences—both the challenges and the moments of connection—shaped me. The anxiety and mistrust that colored my childhood were real, but so was the resilience that carried me through. Whether it was finding a sense of belonging in Cub Scouts, navigating the misunderstandings that led to my removal from the Police Explorers, or adjusting to the upheaval of moving to Golden, I learned to adapt and persevere.

—-

Ever since my adoption, my adoptive father, Berend Sr., had worked in various roles within hospital services. When we lived in Charlevoix, Michigan, he worked in shipping and handling at the local hospital. After our move to Craig, Colorado, he started in a similar role but quickly worked his way up to become the administrator of Memorial Hospital, replacing a man named Frank Weston. Each advancement in his career brought better pay and more stability for our family, but it also meant frequent moves—a reality that was never easy for me or my siblings.

Leaving behind friends was always the hardest part. When we moved to Golden, Colorado, I had to say goodbye to the close-knit group of friends I had made in Craig. However, I was fortunate that some of those friendships endured. Eddie Yeash and Howard Bauer, two of my closest friends from Craig, came to visit me in Golden, and their visits were a reminder of the connections I had built and the support I still had, even from a distance.

In Golden, I made a new friend named Adrian Wells. Adrian was younger than me—around 10 or 11 years old while I was 14—but he quickly became a significant part of my life. In many ways, Adrian filled the void left by the friends I had left behind in

Craig. We spent a lot of time together, and his friendship helped ease the transition to a new place.

I was enrolled at Everett Junior High, a new school with new faces and new challenges. Once again, I found myself navigating the familiar uphill battle of explaining my lack of hair and hearing issues to peers who didn't understand. Starting over was never easy, and the constant need to prove myself in new environments was exhausting. But I wasn't alone in this feeling; I think most children who move frequently can relate to the struggle of leaving behind friends and starting fresh.

Our time in Golden was short-lived. After about a year, my father's career took us to a place that felt like another world: Kotzebue, Alaska, a small community located 35 miles north of the Arctic Circle. To me, it might as well have been another country. Kotzebue was a remote town on the west coast of Alaska, closer to Russia than to most of the United States. The move felt monumental, and I knew it would be a life-changing experience.

We arrived in Kotzebue in December 1988. My father's new role was as the administrator of the PHS Hospital, which later became the Maniilaq Medical Center after being purchased by a local organization. Kotzebue was a unique place, with a population of around 2,500 people during the winter months and up to 5,000 in the summer due to an influx of tourists. The community was predominantly Inupiat Eskimo, with a small percentage of white and Korean residents.

Life in Kotzebue was unlike anything I had ever experienced. The extreme seasons—24 hours of darkness in the winter and 24 hours of daylight in the summer—took some getting used to. But despite the challenges of living in such a remote and harsh environment, I found opportunities to thrive.

One of the most significant opportunities I found in Kotzebue was joining the local EMS service. At just 15 years old, I earned my first medical license, making me one of the youngest medics in the area - or the entire state for that matter. This experience not only gave me a sense of purpose but also helped me make new friends. Kim (Iriuruq) Nay Jr., Jeremy Sharp, Tyson Quinn, and a handful of others became an important part of my life.

Academically, I was also excelling. For the first time, I felt like I was keeping up with—and even surpassing—my peers in certain areas. Some of my classes were held at the Chukchi Campus of the University of Alaska Fairbanks, where I received advanced medical training. These classes were challenging, but they pushed me to grow in ways I hadn't expected.

Socially, I finally felt like I was on equal footing with my peers. The health issues that had plagued me for so long were still present, but they no longer defined me. In Kotzebue, I was seen not as the kid who was different, but as someone who was capable and driven. It was a transformative experience, one that helped me build confidence and a sense of belonging.

Looking back, I can see how each move and each new beginning shaped me. The challenges of leaving behind friends, adjusting to new environments, and navigating the complexities of my health issues taught me resilience. But they also showed me the importance of connection and the power of perseverance.

Kotzebue, in particular, was a turning point for me. It was a place where I found my footing, both academically and socially, and where I began to see myself as more than just a survivor. It was a place where I started to thrive.

Kim Nay Jr., known by his native name Iriuruq—or simply Iri—became the closest friend I had ever had up to that point in my life. Looking back, I can say without hesitation that he was more than a friend; he was like a brother to me. Kim and I spent countless nights at each other's homes, even on school nights, sharing stories, dreams, and the kind of bond that only comes from true camaraderie. Through this friendship, I not only learned more about myself but also began to understand my own sexuality in a way I never had before. Kim would become the first person I ever truly fell in love with.

But our friendship didn't start out the way you might expect. In fact, it began with a conflict—a moment of mischief on my part that could have easily ended in a fight but instead opened the door to one of the most meaningful relationships of my life.

Spring in Kotzebue, Alaska, was unlike spring anywhere else I had lived. The snow didn't melt into the ground as it did in the lower 48 states because of the permafrost—a layer of permanently frozen soil just a foot or so below the surface. Instead, the melting snow pooled into massive puddles that turned the dirt roads into muddy swamps. To manage the standing water, the community used water pumps and long hoses to drain the excess into the Kotzebue Sound, the body of water that bordered the town on three sides.

One day during my first spring in Kotzebue, I was riding my parents' Honda FourTrax ATV through the muddy roads. As I sped down one particularly sloppy stretch, I spotted two individuals trying to navigate on foot along the side of the road. They were doing their best to avoid the deep mud puddles, some of which could reach halfway up a person's knees.

I don't know what came over me that day. Maybe it was boredom, or maybe it was just the kind of impulsive decision that teenagers make without thinking. Whatever the reason, I decided to have a little fun. I revved the engine and sped through the largest puddle I could find, sending a wave of muddy water crashing over the two unsuspecting individuals.

For me, it was just a harmless prank—a moment of innocent mischief. But for Kim and Jeremy, the two people I had just drenched, it was anything but funny. They were soaked, covered in mud, and understandably furious.

A couple of days later, I was confronted by Kim and Jeremy at school. They were ready to fight, and I couldn't blame them. I had been the one to start things, and now I had to face the consequences. But what could have been a physical altercation turned into something entirely different. Instead of throwing punches, we started talking.

I apologized for what I had done, explaining that I hadn't meant any harm. To my surprise, they accepted my apology. What started as a tense confrontation quickly turned into a conversation, and before long, we were laughing about the whole thing. That moment marked the beginning of a friendship that would change my life.

Kim and Jeremy became two of my closest friends, but it was Kim who stood out. He had a warmth and openness that drew people to him, and I felt an immediate connection. Over time, that connection deepened into something more. Kim was the first person I ever truly fell in love with, and though our relationship was complicated, it was also incredibly meaningful.

Kim and I became inseparable. He spent nights at my house, and I spent nights at his. We shared everything—our thoughts, our fears, our dreams. Through Kim, I learned more about myself than I ever had before. He challenged me to be better, to think differently, and to embrace who I was, even when it was hard.

Our friendship wasn't without its challenges. Navigating my feelings for Kim was confusing and sometimes painful, but it was also a crucial part of my journey toward understanding myself. Kim accepted me for who I was, and that acceptance gave me the courage to do the same.

Looking back, it's strange to think that such an important friendship began with a moment of thoughtlessness on my part. If I hadn't splashed Kim and Jeremy that day, if I hadn't made the choice to play a prank, I might never have gotten to know them. And if I hadn't gotten to know Kim, I might never have experienced the kind of connection that shaped me in ways I'm still discovering.

That muddy incident taught me an important lesson: sometimes, the most meaningful relationships come from the most unexpected places. It's a reminder that even our mistakes can lead to something beautiful, if we're willing to learn from them and open ourselves to the possibilities they create.

—-

At 19 years old, I faced one of the hardest goodbyes of my life. Our family was leaving Kotzebue, Alaska, and returning to Michigan. For me, this move was particularly heartbreaking because it meant leaving behind Kim, the closest friend I had ever had. Kim and I had shared so much—laughter, secrets, and a bond that felt unbreakable. Walking away from that friendship felt like leaving a part of myself behind.

The reasons for this move were different from our previous relocations. This time, it wasn't about my father's career advancement; it was about his health. My adoptive father, Berend Sr., had been battling diabetes for years, long before I was even part of the Roeters family. While we were in Alaska, his condition took a dangerous turn. During a doctor's appointment, he was told in no uncertain terms that his health was deteriorating rapidly. The doctor advised him to return to Michigan, to be closer to family and the medical resources he needed.

It was a sobering moment for all of us. My father's health had always been a concern, but now it was a matter of urgency. We packed up our lives in Kotzebue and prepared for the move back to Michigan, knowing that this chapter of our lives was coming to an end.

Before we left Alaska, I had an unexpected encounter with the national spotlight. Through my work with the local EMS service, I was informed by our fire chief that Dr. Bob Arnot, a medical correspondent for 'Good Morning America', might be visiting our hospital. Dr. Arnot was doing a four-day news segment comparing the real medical field in Northwest Alaska to the fictional world of the sitcom 'Northern Exposure'. The chief warned us to be vigilant about protecting patient privacy and to be on the lookout for camera crews.

At the end of 1991, just before we moved, the predicted scenario unfolded. I was on duty when we received a call about a young boy having seizures. We rushed him to the hospital, and as I stepped into the emergency room with my patient, I was met by camera crews attempting to follow us inside. My training kicked in, and I immediately blocked their access, insisting they wait outside until we had permission from the boy's parents.

Unfortunately, the parents were in the hallway and quickly gave their consent for the cameras to film their son. While I respected their decision, I couldn't help but feel conflicted. In my opinion, a minor's medical issues shouldn't be broadcast on national television, regardless of parental permission. But my job was to follow protocol, and I had no choice but to step aside as the cameras rolled.

A few weeks later, in April 1992, my face and the face of my patient were aired on 'Good Morning America'. By then, I was already settling into life in Benzie County, Michigan. The brief moment of fame was a mixed blessing. On one hand, it gave me a sense of recognition when I applied for a position with the Elberta Fire Department. On the other hand, it left me uneasy. I couldn't shake the feeling that the young boy's privacy had been compromised, and it bothered me that his medical crisis had been turned into a spectacle.

Moving back to Michigan was yet another fresh start, and it came with all the usual challenges. Even with the recent notoriety from my appearance on 'Good Morning America', I still had to prove myself in a new community. The familiarity of Michigan was comforting, but it didn't make the transition any easier. I had left behind the people and places that had come to mean so much to me in Alaska, and I wasn't sure how to rebuild that sense of belonging.

For the first time, my older brother Berend Jr. and I lived outside our parents' home. We rented an apartment together, just a mile away from our parents' new house. This arrangement reminded me of the time I had lived with my sister Earlene and her children in Craig, Colorado. It felt like a step toward independence, but it also came with its own set of challenges.

I was no longer in school, and I had to focus on building a life for myself. I found employment, as did Berend Jr., and I joined the local Elberta Fire Department. The fire department became a new anchor in my life, providing a sense of purpose and community. It was a place where I could use the skills I had learned in Alaska and continue to grow as a person.

Looking back, I can see how each move and each new beginning shaped me. The challenges of leaving behind friends, adjusting to new environments, and navigating the complexities of my health issues taught me resilience. But they also showed me the importance of connection and the power of perseverance.

Moving back to Michigan was a turning point in many ways. It marked the end of one chapter and the beginning of another. It was a reminder that life is full of unexpected twists and turns, and that the people we meet along the way can leave a lasting impact on who we become.

Leaving Kotzebue and saying goodbye to Kim was one of the hardest things I've ever had to do. For me, it wasn't just a normal parting of ways; it felt like a tragedy. Kim had been more than a friend—he was a brother, a confidant, and the first person I had ever truly loved. The bond we shared was unlike anything I had experienced before, and walking away from it left a void that took years to fill.

After moving back to Michigan, I struggled with the idea of abandoning my family to return to Alaska. The thought crossed my mind more times than I can count. Part of me wanted to go back, to reclaim the life and the friendships I had left behind. But in the end, I chose to stay near my family. It was a decision I've wrestled with ever since. Some days, I'm grateful for the choice I made. Other days, I can't help but wonder what might have been if I had gone back. Even now, decades later, the question lingers in the back of my mind.

In time, I found a new friend who helped ease the pain of losing Kim. His name was Michael Holtry, and we connected almost immediately. Michael was around my age, and we shared a lot of the same interests. While our friendship never reached the same depth as the one I had with Kim, it was a meaningful and lasting connection. Michael became a source of stability and companionship during a time when I needed it most.

Most of the other friendships I formed in Michigan were with people much older than me, many of whom were members of the Elberta Fire Department. These individuals became mentors and role models, teaching me valuable lessons about life, responsibility, and community. I also continued hunting, a passion I had discovered in Alaska. Now, though, I was hunting with my fellow firefighters, forging bonds over shared experiences in the woods.

It wasn't until I moved back to Michigan that I discovered alcohol—and it quickly took hold of me in ways I hadn't anticipated. What started as a way to unwind and socialize soon became a crutch, something I relied on to numb the pain of losing Kim, the stress of adjusting to a new life, and the grief of losing my father.

Alcohol led me down a dangerous path. It clouded my judgment and led to choices I would later regret—choices that had ripple effects throughout the rest of my life. While this story isn't about those legal troubles, it's important to acknowledge how deeply they affected me. They were a turning point, a reminder of how easily things can spiral out of control when you're not thinking clearly.

Two years after we moved to Michigan, on Memorial Day—just a week after my 21st birthday—my father, Berend William Roeters Sr., passed away. His long battle with diabetes had finally come to an end. Losing him was devastating. He had been a constant presence in my life, a source of strength and stability even during the most turbulent times.

His death hit me hard. In many ways, it felt like the final straw. I was already struggling with the weight of my choices and the lingering pain of leaving Alaska, and his passing pushed me over the edge. I turned to alcohol as a way to cope, but it only made things worse. The grief and guilt I felt were overwhelming, and I made decisions in that haze of emotion that I would later come to regret.

Looking back, I can see how those early years in Michigan shaped me. The loss of my father, the struggles with alcohol, and the mistakes I made were all part of a larger journey—one that taught me hard lessons about responsibility, accountability, and the importance of seeking help when you need it.

But there were also moments of light. Friends like Michael Holtry and the camaraderie I found with the Elberta Fire Department reminded me that I wasn't alone. They showed me that even in the darkest times, there are people who care and who are willing to stand by you.

This is where my story begins to shift: from a young man grappling with loss and poor choices to someone learning to take responsibility for his actions and find a path forward. It's a story of resilience, of picking up the pieces and moving forward, even when the road ahead is uncertain.

In late 1992, shortly after moving back to Michigan from Alaska, something extraordinary happened—I found my biological parents. This moment was years in the making, and it began with a set of court papers that had been tucked away for most of my life. When the Roeters family first fostered me at three and a half years old, they had saved the legal documents detailing my removal from my biological family. My adoptive mother, Mary, had handed me those papers when I was around 12 or 13, telling me I could do whatever I wanted with them. At the time, I didn't think much of it. I stored them with other important documents and forgot about them—until that fateful day in the fall of 1992.

I was cleaning my apartment in Benzie County when I stumbled across the papers. As I picked them up, I noticed the name of the town where I had been born and taken from: Mancelona, Michigan. To my surprise, it was only an hour and a half drive away. The realization hit me like a wave. I had been so close to my roots all along, yet I had never known it.

Tired of cleaning and looking for an excuse to take a break, I decided to act on impulse. I grabbed my keys, hopped into my 1984 LTD station wagon, and drove north to Mancelona. I didn't know what to expect, but I felt a pull I couldn't ignore.

What happened next was nothing short of serendipitous. The moment I arrived in Mancelona, things began to fall into place with an almost surreal ease. It was as if the universe had been waiting for me to take this step. Within hours of arriving in the small town, I found myself face-to-face with my biological parents.

By this time, my biological mother, Sandy, and my biological father, Lionel Cryderman, had divorced and remarried other people. Sandy, who had been the primary reason for my removal from the home as a toddler, had turned her life around. She was now a vibrant, outgoing person who was a joy to be around. For Sandy, reconnecting with me was a deeply emotional experience.

My younger two biological siblings and I were the only children she had ever had, and my return meant she could finally call someone her son again—a title she hadn't used in 16 years.

Lionel, my biological father, had also remarried. His wife, Tammy, was a kind and loving woman who embraced all of Lionel's children, regardless of who their mothers were. Lionel himself had nine children with five or six different women, but he was a devoted father despite his own health struggles, which were primarily cardiac-related. He had always been protective of his children, and his joy at seeing me again was palpable.

Both Sandy and Lionel were thrilled to have me back in their lives. For me, it was a whirlwind of emotions—joy, curiosity, and a sense of belonging I hadn't realized I was missing.

My reconnection with my biological family didn't stop with my parents. I also met siblings and cousins I had never known existed. The experience was overwhelming in the best possible way. For a while, I even moved to Mancelona and lived with my biological grandmother, Shirley Williams, in her little yellow house next to the first gas station you see when entering the town.

Living in Mancelona gave me the chance to immerse myself in the family I had lost so many years ago. I spent time with Sandy, Lionel, and my extended family, learning about their lives and sharing my own story. It was a time of healing and discovery, but it didn't last long. Eventually, I moved back to Benzie County, where I continued my friendship with Michael Holtry and rebuilt my life there.

Michael had become a cornerstone of my life in Michigan. Our friendship wasn't as intense as the bond I had shared with Kim, but it was steady and reliable. Michael was someone I could count on, and he played a significant role in helping me navigate the complexities of reconnecting with my biological family and adjusting to life in Michigan.

When I eventually moved back to Mancelona for a second time, Michael came with me. Our friendship was strong enough to withstand the changes, and we even ventured up to the Upper Peninsula of Michigan together for a while. It was during this time that Michael met a girlfriend and had a daughter, further solidifying his own roots in the state.

Finding my biological family was a pivotal moment in my life. It filled in gaps I hadn't even realized were there and gave me a deeper understanding of where I came from. But it also raised new questions about identity, belonging, and the choices we make.

Reconnecting with Sandy and Lionel was bittersweet. While I was grateful to have them back in my life, I couldn't help but wonder how things might have been different if I had grown up with them. At the same time, I knew that my life with the Roeters family had shaped me in ways I wouldn't trade for anything.

This chapter of my life was about more than just finding my biological family; it was about finding myself. It was about understanding that family isn't just about blood—it's about the connections we forge and the love we share, whether through birth, adoption, or friendship.

As I reflect on this period of my life, I'm struck by how much I've grown. The journey from Alaska to Michigan, from Kim to Michael, from the Roeters family to my biological parents, has been one of resilience and self-discovery. It hasn't always been easy, but it has been worth it.

This is where this part of my story ends—a story of reconnection, healing, and the enduring power of family in all its forms. But it's also the beginning of a new chapter, one that will take me even further on the path to understanding who I am and where I belong.

This is my legacy. And it is only the beginning.

Chapter 2

The door creaks as I open it—not just the physical one, but the one in my mind. A sound like rusted hinges giving way after decades of disuse. Memories flood in, sharp and unrelenting, carried on a current of antiseptic and childhood fear. Fifty-one years of life, of drifting between Colorado's snow-capped mountains, Alaska's frozen silence, Texas's sweltering sprawl, and Florida's humid glare. But geography never mattered. No matter where I went, my body carried the same invisible scars.

PBB poisoning. Those three letters still taste bitter on my tongue, like licking a battery.

I was four years old when the Roeters family took me in—a child already marked by something no one understood. The hearing aids came first, bulky beige contraptions strapped to my ears like relics from a forgotten war. Then the baldness: a smooth, hairless scalp that made teachers whisper and kids ask if I was "a cancer patient" or "an alien." The truth, it turned out, was stranger than anything their playground imaginations could conjure.

Doctors' offices became my second home. The smell of rubbing alcohol and wilted magazines. The cold pinch of needles sliding into veins, glass vials filling with ruby-red blood under fluorescent lights. But the worst was the muscle test. After the syringes came the ache—deep, bone-deep, as if my body were punishing me for surrendering what little it had left.

And the spinal tap? That was the day I learned fear could be a physical thing. The room was too bright, all white walls and cold steel. The smell of rubbing alcohol was so strong it made my eyes water. Mrs. Roeter held my hand, but her grip was tight with her own fear. The doctor's voice was a low murmur, 'Just a small pinch, son, then you need to hold very, very still.' But the hands that turned me on my side were not asking; they were placing me. I felt the cold swipe of the iodine, a shocking yellow circle on my skin. Then the pressure, a deep, wrong pressure as the needle searched for a space that should never be touched. And then it came—not a pinch, but a white-hot wire, a live current of pure wrongness threading down the core of me, down my leg, screaming 'this should not be happening.' I didn't scream out loud. I held my breath until spots danced in the white ceiling, my whole world narrowed to that single, violating wire of pain.

The MRIs were almost a relief. At least in that claustrophobic tube, with its mechanical screams, no one could see me cry.

School was its own kind of laboratory—a place where children distilled cruelty into casual questions. "Why don't you have eyebrows?" "Your ears look like robot parts." I learned to laugh it off, to lean into the caricature. If I was the "bald kid with radar ears," fine—I'd be the funny bald kid. I remember one birthday party, a classmate pointing at my plate of fruit while everyone else ate pizza. "What's wrong with you?" he'd sneered. I'd forced a grin, puffing out my chest. "Superior genetics. Pizza is for mere mortals." They laughed. I spent the rest of the party with a knot in my stomach, the ghost of milk allergy cramps twisting in my gut. Humor was armor. Scouts, firefighting, the police explorers program—those were my escapes. For a few hours, I could pretend I was more than a diagnosis.

But the shadow followed. It was in my ribs, which popped like dry twigs wrestling with my brother. It was in my teeth, which chipped from nothing, from just existing too hard. The doctors called it "brittle." I called it betrayal. At sixteen, while other boys bragged about stubble and growth spurts, my body stayed stubbornly, eerily smooth. No armpit hair. No chest hair. Just... blank skin. The doctors shrugged. "Delayed development." The kids sneered. "Freak."

I called it survival.

—-

In 1992, I was living in my first home as a young adult in Elberta, Michigan. It was a small place I shared with my older adoptive brother. On a day off work, during a fit of spring cleaning, I found myself sitting on the edge of my bed with a cardboard box of childhood keepsakes in my lap.

My adoptive parents were awesome parents. And, unknowingly, they had given me the breadcrumb trail I needed. When I was about ten, my adoptive mother decided I had the right to hold the court papers from my adoption. They'd been in a manila envelope, tucked away for years.

That day, for the first time, I didn't just glance at them. I read them. The words were dry, legal, but they held a thunderous truth. The community I was taken from, the family I couldn't remember—they were only about an hour and a half away.

My heart raced. I dropped the papers, ran to my car, and fumbled for my paper folding map. Spreading it on the hood of my 1994 Ford LTD station wagon, my finger traced the route north. Mancelona, Michigan. It was right there.

I was tired from cleaning. My mind was made up. I was done for the day. With no plan other than the name on the papers, I got in my car and headed towards Antrim County.

The drive was a blur of nervous energy. As the forests closed in around me, halfway between Kalkaska and Mancelona, my body grew both numb and buzzing with anxiety. Who would I ask? What if they slammed the door in my face? What if they didn't remember me? What if I had to say the words, "Hi, I'm your son"?

It was almost scary how easily I found them. I asked two people in town about my biological last name. Both pointed me in the same direction. On the third stop, I was standing on my biological grandmother's porch.

The reunion was emotional, a whirlwind of tears and hugs. My two biological parents, who had divorced, came together because I had come back. But beneath the joy, there was tension. Aunts and uncles had negative things to say, finger-pointing about who was at fault for me and my two younger siblings being taken away. My biological mother had drug issues when I was a toddler, though they were long gone by then.

But then, something else happened. In conversations with my newfound family, a topic I never brought up was voluntarily offered: the 1973 PBB cattle poisoning. They spoke of it freely, a known shadow over the region. It was local gossip to them, a tragedy that happened to farmers and their cows.

But to me, combined with the map of my own health issues, these mentions of PBB ceased to be just stories. They became a trail. The first clue in a mystery written on my own body. And I had no choice but to start following it.

—-

The moment the puzzle pieces snapped together, the world didn't just shift—it made sense for the first time. The allergies. The baldness. The bones that snapped like dry twigs. It had a name. PBB—polybrominated biphenyl. A chemical accident in Michigan's dairy farms, poisoning the food chain, slipping into mothers' milk, into me. The Roeters had suspected, but how do you tell a child their body is a battleground for corporate negligence?

The realization was a double-edged sword. Relief—finally, an answer. But also a cold, settling rage. All those years of pain, of otherness, reduced to a footnote in a medical report. I'd been a statistic before I'd even known my own name.

This new understanding cast my entire childhood in a different, harsher light. I wasn't just a sick kid. I was a poisoned one. The story of my biological siblings, Tina and Lonnie, was never just mine. We were three strands of the same poisoned thread, woven into separate lives but bound by something none of us could see.

When the Roeters took me in, they did something rare: they kept the door open. Not just for me, but for Tina and Lonnie too. Most families would've severed those ties. Mine didn't. Maybe they sensed we'd need each other someday.

Tina was the middle child, her scalp as smooth as mine, her body just as rebellious. Where my allergies attacked my stomach, hers flared on her skin—angry red patches bandaged under wigs. "It's fine," she'd say, her voice tight. But it wasn't. None of it was.

Lonnie, the youngest, seemed untouched at first. No baldness, no rashes. But poison doesn't always announce itself. His adoptive family ignored the whispers, just like Tina's. Denial was easier than digging for answers.

Years later, when I found Lonnie in Michigan—sixteen, angry, and clashing with his adoptive father—I became more than a brother. I became his guardian. Overnight, we were a family of fractured pieces, trying to fit together edges that didn't match. It was a desperate attempt to create a shelter from a storm we didn't yet fully understand.

The storm, however, was only gathering strength.

—-

Thirty-nine years old. That's how old I was when my body finally screamed loud enough for the world to hear.

One moment, standing. The next—collapse. A lightning strike of wrongness searing down my right side. Arm dead. Chest numb. The floor rushing up to meet me.

The diagnosis: stroke at 39.

Doctors muttered about anomalies. Bad luck. Rare case.

But I knew.

We all knew.

The right side of my body became a stranger. My arm—once strong enough to break doors—now hung limp, a useless weight. Muscles in my chest withered as if the stroke had siphoned them away.

I learned new words:

· Hemiparesis. Weakness on one side.

· Neuropathy. Nerves screaming at nothing.

· TIA. The silent time bomb in my brain.

Then, April 2020—another stroke. This one brought seizures, my body convulsing like a downed power line. The scans showed the truth: my veins, frail and aged decades beyond the rest of me.

Premature aging.

Of course.

PBB doesn't just poison you. It erodes you.

Insurance companies spat numbers at me. Too expensive. Pre-existing. Denied.

Disability? The word tasted like surrender.

My adoptive parents' voices echoed: "You earn what you get."

So I adapted. Typing one-handed. Relearning balance. Ignoring stares when my arm spasmed mid-conversation.

This isn't pride. It's defiance.

PBB stole enough from me. It doesn't get my dignity too.

—-

They told me strokes were for old men. For smokers. For the unlucky.

But I was poisoned before I could walk.

Every seizure, every numb limb, every doctor's frown—they're not just symptoms. They're evidence.

And I'm still here to testify.

This book isn't just my story. It's a ledger. A tally of what was taken—and what they failed to destroy.

The door's open now.

And I'm not just walking through.

I'm kicking it down.

—-

Looking back at a lifetime of health battles—some I've carried since birth—one truth burns brighter than the rest: most kids who dealt with half of what I did didn't make it.

Dying was never on my agenda.

Not when my ribs cracked like eggshells during a playground tumble. Not when my veins collapsed under the weight of too many blood draws. Not even when doctors exchanged those silent, grave looks over my charts, their pens hovering over words like "failure to thrive." My body was a warzone, but surrender wasn't in my DNA.

When I was 11, I met Jason Gaes—or at least, his story. A kid my age who'd stared down cancer at nine and won. His parents made a documentary about it: "You Don't Have to Die."

I didn't have cancer. But I had fear—thick, choking fear—every time a white coat walked into the room. Because I knew what came next: needles, cold stethoscopes, the metallic taste of panic as another test ripped answers from my body.

Jason's face on that grainy VHS tape was a lifeline. Here was a boy who'd swallowed radiation like it was candy, who'd lost his hair just like me, but not to some invisible poison—to a battle he'd chosen to fight. And he'd won.

Watching him grin through baldness, through scars, through pain, did something to me: It made my suffering feel like a choice, too. Not the pain itself—but how I carried it.

So I stopped cringing when the IV went in. Stopped crying when the spinal tap needle kissed my spine. I'd clench my jaw and think: Jason did this. So can I.

PBB wrecked lives. It turned my childhood into a medical footnote and my body into a cautionary tale. But it failed at one thing: breaking me.

Every snapped bone taught me how to mend. Every cruel nickname honed my humor into a weapon. Every doctor's doubt fueled a stubbornness that's outlasted every prognosis.

Jason is gone now. Passed away for reasons unrelated to the cancer he fought as a child. But the boy I never met face-to-face—the nine-year-old who stared into a camera with bald head and blazing eyes in that documentary—he's still with me. His voice, scratchy from the VHS tape we wore thin from rewinding, lives in my bones: "You don't have to die."

For over forty years, I've carried his example like a talisman. Not because he was extraordinary, but because he proved something I needed to believe: A child's body can be at war and still choose to survive.

—-

Last year, I found the registry.

A crumpled webpage, buried in some corporate server, listing the names of those affected by PBB poisoning. The company that maintains it—the same one that swapped fire retardant for cattle feed in '73—treats it like a footnote. No updates. No outreach. Just a digital graveyard of the poisoned.

I added my name anyway.

Not for them. For the others like me—the ones still searching for answers, still rubbing absentmindedly at the patches of skin where hair never grew, still wondering why their bones snap like dry twigs at fifty. For the mothers who drank the milk and passed the poison to their babies. For the generations after us, whose fat cells still hoard this chemical curse like a time capsule.

Our bodies are the evidence they couldn't burn.

—-

Ron Howard's Bitter Harvest laid it bare: the Michigan farmer watching his cows stagger and die, their milk laced with a chemical they never named on the news. The government's response? A shrug. A payout. A paper trail swept into filing cabinets.

But the movie didn't show the real aftermath.

It didn't show the children like me—adopted out, scattered across states, our symptoms dismissed as "bad luck." It didn't show the mothers who nursed infants with poison milk, their wombs later expelling stillborns with PBB-laced livers. It didn't show the grandchildren born decades later, their DNA already scribbled with errors no one could explain.

This wasn't an accident. It was a mass poisoning—and the cover-up was clinical.

PBB doesn't just harm. It inherits.

It nestles in fat cells, leaching into breastmilk, crossing placentas. It rewires hormones, stunts growth, turns bones to glass. And when the original victims die? It jumps to their children. Their grandchildren. A chain reaction of suffering with no expiration date.

I've met them—the next generation. The teens with my same bald patches, the toddlers allergic to sunlight. Their parents hand me ultrasound photos like affidavits: "Look. It's happening again."

And I lived it. Although I was afraid that one or both of my children would wind up with health issues involving PBB like I grew up with, it would turn out that it was only my son. He needed hearing aids in his teenage years, a bitter echo of my own childhood. And he had childhood cancer. Seeing him face that was perhaps one of the scariest moments of my life—a terrifying glimpse of my own past and a painful proof that my legacy was now his.

The government called it a "localized agricultural incident."

But poison doesn't respect borders. Or apologies. Or time.

They wanted us silent.

Wanted the farmers to take the checks and disappear. Wanted kids like me to die quietly in foster homes, our symptoms chalked up to "bad genes." Wanted the world to forget.

But Jason taught me this: Survival is a story. And stories outlive their tellers.

So I'll say it loud—for the boy on the VHS tape, for the names on that forgotten registry, for the babies born poisoned tomorrow:

We remember.

We're still here.

And we're not done.

—-

The first time I held proof they'd known, my hands shook so badly I nearly dropped the page.

It was 2017, in the basement archives of a Michigan public health department. A clerk had led me past shelves of moldering ledgers to a banker's box labeled Livestock Feed Incident, 1973-76. Inside, sandwiched between invoices for condemned cattle, I found it:

MEMORANDUM

To: State Epidemiologist

From: Dr. L.H. (redacted)

Date: May 14, 1974

Subject: Human Exposure Concerns

*Preliminary fat biopsies from farm families show PBB retention at 50-300 ppm. Of particular concern are the children, who exhibit:

· Delayed skeletal maturation

· Persistent dermal lesions

· Thyroid abnormalities*

Recommend immediate breastmilk testing for lactating mothers. Long-term monitoring advised due to compound's lipophilic persistence.

The paper smelled of vinegar—a preservative for disintegrating ink. I traced the faded typewriter text with one finger, my own thyroid scar throbbing under my collar. They'd known. Known while I was still a bald four-year-old sucking down contaminated milk from a Roeters family sippy cup.

The clerk coughed. "You can't remove originals, but we have a photocopier."

I stood there, paralyzed. This single page explained more about my body than 19 years of doctors' guesses. Yet someone had stamped CONFIDENTIAL across it and buried it for 43 years.

Getting the rest of the story required dancing with bureaucrats who'd mastered the art of no.

Attempt 1 (2018):

"All records related to PBB human health assessments, 1973-1980."

The FDA's response:"No responsive documents located."

Attempt 2 (2019):

A narrower request:"Meeting minutes between Michigan Dept. of Agriculture and Chemical Corp X, 1974."

They sent 300 pages—280 fully redacted,the rest so heavily blacked out they looked like abstract art. One legible fragment:

"...cost of livestock compensation estimated at $3M, far less than recall..."

Attempt 3 (2020):

I hired a lawyer.Six months later, we got the crown jewel: internal memos from the feed mill where the mix-up started.

"Workers noted the FireMaster bags smelled 'funny' but assumed formula change. No lot numbers recorded."

Translation: A multi-generational poisoning began because someone couldn't be bothered to label toxic waste.

The most damning evidence often hid in handwritten notes. In the margins of a 1975 USDA report, some anonymous official had scribbled:

"If we admit fetal risk, opens door to lawsuits. Stick to cattle."

I found it tucked between minutes about indemnifying farmers for dead cows. No mention of the stillbirths piling up in rural clinics. No autopsies for the infants born with livers the size of walnuts.

That's when I realized: We weren't just poisoned. We were erased.

In 1976, the CDC proposed a longitudinal study of exposed children. The plan? Track 200 adopted kids like me for "developmental anomalies."

The funding vanished after Chemical Corp X donated $2M to a senator's re-election campaign.

I tracked down the study's lead researcher before he died. Over whiskey in his retirement home, he spat:

"They told us 'focus on the cows.' So we did. And you kids? You became statistical noise."

His hands trembled with Parkinson's—a condition now linked to PBB exposure. The irony wasn't lost on either of us.

That night, I spread the documents across my kitchen table—FOIA rejections, lab reports, the single unredacted memo.

My cat batted at a page, leaving claw marks over the words thyroid abnormalities.

I stared at my reflection in the blackened window. Somewhere out there, other orphans of the poisoning were still searching for answers.

Tomorrow, I'd begin testing the one piece of evidence they couldn't redact:

My own body.

November 2018 - University of Michigan Toxicology Lab

The biopsy needle was colder than I expected.

Deep breath now," said Dr. Chen as she slid the 14-gauge harpoon into the soft flesh above my hipbone. The crunch as it pierced my fat layer sounded like teeth biting into celery. Somewhere in that yellow glob of tissue—the same stubborn padding that had survived every childhood steroid treatment and adult starvation diet—were the molecules that had shaped my life.

The vial filled with a viscous, buttery substance. My blood looked almost pink against it.

"Congratulations," Chen deadpanned. "You're officially the most interesting patient this month."

Three weeks later, the results arrived in a PDF so dense with acronyms it might as well have been hieroglyphics. One number leaped out:

PBB-153: 4,217 ppb

The safety threshold for Michigan soil contamination was 20 ppb. My fat carried 200 times that.

—-

A MAP WRITTEN IN SCARS

I spread the lab report next to my childhood medical records on the motel bed. The correlations lined up like evidence tags at a crime scene:

Year Symptom PBB Mechanism

1976 (Age 4) Bald patches, hearing loss Bromine disruption of keratin/hair follicles; cochlear degeneration

1987 (Age 15) Failed puberty Endocrine disruption - mimics/ blocks testosterone

1999 (Age 27) "Unexplained" bone fractures Calcium leaching from bones; collagen malformation

2012 (Age 39) Stroke Accelerated atherosclerosis from vascular inflammation

The most damning note came from a 1983 endocrinologist: "Patient's condition resembles experimental animal models exposed to halogenated hydrocarbons."

They'd known. For forty fucking years.

Dr. Chen invited me to view my fat cells under the microscope. The PBBs didn't glow or pulse—they just sat there, dull brown blobs nestled against my lipids like ticks.

"Here's the scary part," she said, switching to an electron micrograph. "See these pockmarks? That's where the molecules bonded permanently to cell membranes. Your body didn't store this poison. It became the poison."

She showed me a normal fat cell for comparison—smooth as a pearl.

Mine looked like a grenade had gone off inside.

The university kept requesting "additional samples." They took:

· Hair: Strands still carried traces 30 years after my last exposure

· Breath: Exhaled gases revealed ongoing liver metabolism of PBBs

· Baby teeth: Dug from my mother's keepsake box, their growth rings showed contamination in utero

Each test felt like an archeological dig through my own flesh. The final blow came when they analyzed a sliver of my rib bone—removed during a 2007 surgery:

"PBB-153 detected in osteocytes (bone cells). Half-life estimates exceed 70 years."

Translation: I would die with this inside me.

They tested my niece's baby teeth next. Same concentric rings of contamination.

When the genetic counselor said "epigenetic inheritance," my sister collapsed into the kind of sobbing that comes from realizing your womb was never safe.

That night, I dreamt of FireMaster bags splitting open, their amber flakes swirling into milk bottles, IV bags, amniotic fluid.

I woke gasping at 3 AM and drove to the 24-hour Walmart. In the baby aisle, I ran my fingers over formula cans, checking labels for ingredients no one would list.

Somewhere out there, another child was drinking their future.

—

Mancelona Public Library, Michigan - March 2019

The microfilm machine smelled like burning dust and old pennies. As I scrolled through the Antrim County News from 1975, the births and deaths columns told twin stories:

January 3: "Born to Daniel and Marie Whitcomb, a daughter, 5 lbs 2 oz. Died January 4."

March 17:"Stillborn son delivered to Robert and Ellen Visser at Mercy Hospital."

June 9:"Infant daughter of James and Lori Pearson passed peacefully in her sleep."

Page after page, summer to winter, the same pattern: clusters of neonatal deaths with causes like "failure to thrive" or simply blank. The librarian hovered behind me.

"You're the third person this month looking at those," she said. "Health department intern was here just last week."

I turned so fast the film reel rattled. "What intern?"

She shrugged. "Some girl taking notes. Said she was working on a... whatchacallit... cluster study?"

The hairs on my neck stood up. Someone was finally counting.

Ruth Anne Miller's hands trembled as she flipped through her 1974 birthing records. At 89, her memory fogged on names but never numbers.

"Normal years, maybe three, four stillbirths," she said. "That summer? Twenty-two between May and August. Mostly farm families."

Her ledger entries read like horror haikus:

"Baby Boy Henderson - born blue, no breath. Liver enlarged 3x normal."

"Baby Girl Laughlin - lived 6 hours. Skin peeled like old wallpaper."

She paused at one page, finger resting on a coffee stain. "This one... the mother kept screaming 'It's not shaped right!' We wrapped it quick before she could see."

The health department's official report: "Congenital anomalies - no further action required."

Cross-referencing death certificates with adoption records revealed a darker pattern. For every dead infant, there were three like me—sick children quietly shipped out of state.

I tracked down seven through foster care databases:

· Case #A-1142: Boy, 3 yrs old. Chronic seizures. Adopted by family in Colorado, 1976. Died age 12 (status epilepticus).

· Case #B-7719: Girl, 18 mos. Alopecia totalis. Adopted by family in Texas. Last known address: psychiatric facility, 2004.

· Case #C-3358: Me.

The social worker who processed my file in '75 was still alive in a Traverse City nursing home. She remembered the instructions:

"They told us not to ask about birth family medical history. Said it would 'prejudice adoptive parents.'"

Her fingernails dug into the wheelchair arms. "We were baby brokers for damaged goods."

The University of Michigan's lost study files contained one chilling photo: twelve children lined up for a 1982 "developmental assessment." All bald. All small for their age. All wearing hearing aids.

I'm the only one still alive.

The researcher's notes:

"Subject #7 - Advanced bone age but arrested puberty. Parents report 'glass bones.' Recommend endocrine consult."

That was Tina.She overdosed at 24.

"Subject #12 - Violent outbursts, self-mutilation. Possible neurotoxicity."

Lonnie.Prison by 19.

Our blood samples, labeled with peeling stickers, still sit in a Lansing storage freezer. Nobody ever followed up.

At a 2020 PBB survivors' meeting, I met Carrie Ann Beukema—born six months after the contamination peaked. Her medical chart mirrored mine stroke for stroke. When she lifted her shirt, the same surgical scars laddered her ribs.

"We're mirrors," she whispered. Then showed me her daughter's ultrasound: the same speckled shadows on the liver that had haunted my niece's scans.

The poison didn't just persist. It replicated.

That night, I dreamed of the ghost children again. They stood in a hospital nursery, pressing tiny hands against glass smeared with milk residue.

When I woke, my email pinged—a message from the health department intern:

"Found something you should see. Meet me at the old feed mill. Bring a flashlight."

—-

June 2021 - VFW Hall #317, Cadillac, Michigan

The folding chairs squeaked as twenty-three of us arranged ourselves in a lopsided circle. Bald heads. Wheelchairs. A symphony of cane taps and arrhythmic heart monitors. Carrie Ann passed around a Tupperware of chocolate chip cookies she couldn't eat (celiac from gut damage) and a sign-in sheet with a new column:

"Symptoms in Children/Grandchildren:"

- "My son's teeth crumbled by age 4"
- "Granddaughter born without tear ducts"
- "Twins both autistic, seizures started at 18 months"

Dr. Chen knelt by an IV pole, drawing blood from a farmer's leathery arm. "This isn't a support group anymore," she said. "It's a field study."

The label on the first vial: PATIENT ZERO - SURVIVOR COHORT.

We armed ourselves like guerilla researchers:

· $29 Amazon centrifuges for separating serum

· Smuggled biopsy punches from a veterinary supply store

· A shared Google Drive labeled "Livestock Incident Follow-Up"

The health department intern—Maya, a 22-year-old biochemistry student—showed up with binders of stolen records. Her hands shook as she distributed copies.

"These prove they tracked us," she said.

The documents:

1. A 1982 memo listing "high-risk adoptees" by case number (mine circled in red)

2. Lab results from a never-published CDC study showing PBB in our breastmilk

3. A budget line item: "Contingency for genetic liability claims - $1.2M"

They'd known we'd reproduce. Known the poison would outlive them.

Maya's discovery in the old feed mill wasn't documents—it was samples.

"Behind the asbestos insulation," she whispered, shining her phone light on rows of mason jars. Each held a fetal specimen floating in yellowed formalin. The labels read:

STILLBORN #4 - QUARANTINED HERD, JUNE 1974

NEONATAL LIVER - DAIRY FARMER'S CHILD

No names. No death certificates. Just biological evidence hidden like moonshine.

When we tested the liver tissue, the PBB levels were 900 times higher than anything recorded in cattle.

The voicemail came at 3:17 AM:

"It's Jim from the health lab. I... I processed those baby autopsies. They made us sign nondisclosures. The liver weights alone should've—" A choking sound. "Christ, the livers were calcified like rocks. Meet me at the boat launch tomorrow. Bring a recorder."

We never got the recording. Jim's obituary ran two days later: "Unexpected complications from a long illness."

His widow handed me a napkin at the funeral. On it, scribbled in shaky Sharpie:

"Check Lot #1147. They rebranded."

Lot #1147 led to a factory in Ohio. Same chemical company, new name. Same amber powder, new label: FireShield XP™ - Now With 30% Less Bioaccumulation!

The safety data sheet listed the active ingredient: "Proprietary brominated polymer."

Dr. Chen ran the mass spec. The readout flashed:

PBB-209: Modified side chain, same core structure

"They didn't stop making it," she said. "They just made it harder to trace."

At our last meeting, we lined up the evidence:

1. 48 survivors with matching epigenetic markers

2. 17 second-generation victims showing identical symptoms

3. 3 jars of stolen tissue samples proving intergenerational transfer

4. Most residents of Northern Michigan have elevated levels of PBB in their fat cells as of today as a result of the 1973 poisoning.

Carrie Ann projected a map onto the VFW's stained wallpaper. Red dots marked every cancer cluster within 50 miles of a FireShield plant.

"Statistically impossible," whispered the retired math teacher in our group. Then louder: "Statistically impossible!"

We all heard the unspoken truth: They were still doing it. Still lying. Still counting on us to die quietly.

The night before filing the class-action lawsuit, I dreamed of Jim standing waist-deep in Lake Michigan, holding a jar labeled STILLBORN #5.

"Keep counting," he said, pushing it toward me.

When I woke, the first subpoenas were already printing.

The door's open now. And I'm not just walking through.

I'm kicking it down.

Chapter 3

I remember that first day being brought to my adopted family. Memory is a strange, fragmented thing-especially when it stretches back to early childhood. Some details are soft at the edges, blurred by time and the simple fact that I was so very young. Others are etched with a startling clarity, as if lit by a sudden bolt of lightning against a dark sky. I remember the drive, a long stretch of countryside road unfurling like a tired gray ribbon through northern Michigan. The trees were mostly bare; it must have been late fall. The world outside the car window was a wash of browns and muted greens, the sky a flat, pale sheet of cloud.

The vehicle itself stands out in my mind. It was a sedan belonging to the social worker, a woman whose name I've since lost, but whose faint scent of lavender and polyester has lingered in some sensory corner of my brain. What fascinated my young mind were the locks and windows. This car had the earliest, most modest levels of electronic buttons-perhaps among the first of their kind on vehicles in 1977. A small, square button you pressed to lock the doors with a heavy thunk. A switch, not a crank, to lower the window with a slow, electric hum. To my memory, every other vehicle I'd been in had hand-operated handles for rolling the windows up and down, or those stiff, chrome knobs you pulled up to unlock the door. Those tiny, futuristic controls felt like magic. At 52 years old, it's amazing what you can look back at and remember-the minor, mechanical details that somehow symbolize a crossing from one world into another.

We pulled into a gravel driveway. The house was white, two stories, with a wide front porch that seemed to wrap itself around the structure in a tired embrace. There was a barn off to the side, red paint peeling in long, elegant strips. The social worker turned off the engine, and the sudden silence felt heavy. She gave me a practiced, gentle smile. "This is going to be a good place," she said, a phrase I would hear many times in many variations. We got out, the gravel crunching under our shoes. She took my small hand in hers, and we walked up the three wooden steps to the porch. Before she could even knock, the front door swung open.

And a goat ran out.

It happened so fast. A blur of wiry white fur, a flash of curved horn, a startled baaaa that was more indignation than alarm. It barreled between us, nearly knocking me off my feet. I stumbled back, my heart a frantic drum against my ribs. I'd seen pictures of goats, maybe, but this was a living, breathing, charging creature, smelling of hay and animal musk. It was an experience I had never had, and in my already overwhelmed state, it felt less like a welcome and more like an ambush.

Mrs. Roeters appeared in the doorway a second later, a hand flying to her mouth. "Oh, for heaven's sake! Washday, you get back here!" she called after the retreating goat, but it was already disappearing around the side of the house. She shook her head, then turned her attention to us. Her expression shifted from mild exasperation to a warm, enveloping kindness.

Mrs. Roeters, as she stood at the door, looking at the social worker and then looking down at me, didn't realize how my small mind was traumatized by the goat nearly running me over. To her, it was a daily farm mishap. To me, it was the chaotic prologue to my new life. Nothing less, she invited both of us into the home.

"Please, come in, come in. Pay no mind to that escape artist," she said, her voice as warm as her smile. And what a smile it was.

It reached her eyes, which were a soft, hazel color, crinkling at the corners. It wasn't a smile of pity, nor one of forced cheer. It was a smile that seemed to show she was a very understanding human being, someone who had seen frayed edges before and wasn't afraid of them. It was a bit of reassurance that was profoundly inviting, especially compared to my previous, fractured experiences with adults before this moment in my life.

The inside of the house was a testament to busy, loving chaos. The living room was cluttered but clean, dominated by a large, worn sofa and the smell of baked bread and wood smoke. Toys were scattered in one corner, a basket of laundry waited to be folded in another. She led us to a comfortable, overstuffed armchair patterned with faded roses. "Would you like to sit here, sweetie?" she asked me. I nodded, mute, and climbed into its embrace. The fabric was soft and smelled faintly of old pipe tobacco.

It would be during the conversation that Mrs. Roeters had with the social worker, as I just sat in that comfortable chair, that my attention would be pulled away. The adults spoke in low, serious tones about paperwork, adjustments, and "transition periods." I let the words wash over me, a meaningless adult hum, and stared out the window. That's when I saw it: a baby-blue colored Volkswagen Beetle bouncing up the driveway, kicking up a small plume of dust. It parked beside our sedan.

Moments later, the front door opened again, letting in a burst of cool air. A gentleman with a bright, bushy red beard, like a friendly explosion of copper wire, filled the doorway. His cheeks were wind-chapped, and he wore a thick flannel shirt. His eyes, a startling blue, scanned the room and immediately landed on me.

"Well, hello there," he boomed, his voice cheerful and large. He didn't hesitate. Within his arms he held a stuffed beaver animal, its brown plush fur worn soft. He crossed the room in two strides and knelt before my chair, bringing himself to my eye level. He didn't offer it to the social worker or his wife first. He immediately handed it to me. "I heard we might be having a new explorer joining us. Every explorer needs a companion. This is Bucky. He's been waiting for you."

The gesture was so direct, so unadorned with ceremony, that I took the toy without thinking. Its softness was an immediate comfort in my hands. As he immediately engaged in conversation with Mrs. Roeters and the social worker, his eyes and attention kept flicking back to me. He'd nod along to something the social worker said, but he'd wink at me. He'd listen to his wife, but he'd smile in my direction. It was as if I were silently included in the circle, not as a subject of discussion, but as a participant.

Within just a few hours, the paperwork signed and promises made, the social worker was gone. The lavender scent faded from the air, replaced by the solid, real smells of the farmhouse. And I was quickly learning about the older children that lived in the home. Their names were recited to me like a new, important list: Berend Jr.-at the time known as just Junior-was the only biological son, lanky and quiet. Brian, with watchful eyes. Scott, who seemed to vibrate with restless energy. And Earlene, whose presence felt different, calmer, like a deep, still pool.

My communication skills lacked a lot of understanding with those within the household. Words felt slippery, and sentences often came out in a confused jumble or didn't come out at all. I had a language inside my head, but translating it into speech felt like trying to catch minnows with my bare hands. But somehow, I fitted in. The chaos of the farmhouse had its own rhythm, and my silent observation became a kind of participation. Those communication skills-or lack thereof-would cause some issues. A misheard instruction, a frustrated tear when I couldn't explain a simple need. But through it, my new foster family would find a way to communicate with me. Mrs. Roeters became an expert at reading my face. Mr. Roeters used gestures and patient repetition. Even though, to them, it must have been like learning a new, cryptic language, they kept trying.

My foster family, who lived in Ellsworth, Michigan, owned a small farm just outside of the community. In reality, it wasn't very far from my biological family that I'd just been removed from. The same pine trees, the same chill off Lake Michigan, the same dirt roads. Yet it felt like a different planet. However, between the time from my biological family and my new family, there had been other foster homes. Brief, shadowy stops in other houses with other kind-but-weary faces. But I had been tracked down, by my biological father, and forcefully removed from those foster homes and taken out of the country to Canada multiple times. These were journeys of fear and confusion, of night drives and hushed arguments. After being found, and relocated back to northern Michigan by Canadian law enforcement and the FBI-a fact I would only piece together decades later from cold court documents-I was now in my current predicament: being refostered into the home of the Roeters family. They were told, I later learned, that I needed stability above all else. A port in a storm I had been too young to understand I was caught in.

Still today, at the age of 52, I look back and find that it's weird that even though I remember that first day with this family—the goat, the blue Beetle, the stuffed beaver-I don't hold a single memory of a single day before this. It's as if my life started on that porch. It's odd how the human brain works. A single organ in your body designed to protect you from everything, even, perhaps especially, the memory of your own past. A self-erasing chalkboard for the soul's too-painful equations. A portion of what I just wrote was based not on memory, but on court documents and legal work that I later discovered in my adult life, files that told a story my mind had chosen to forget.

One of my most vivid memories in that house in Ellsworth, Michigan, would be the winter storm of 1978. The Great Blizzard. While some of those memories are vague, painted in the monochrome of white and dark, one scene is crystal clear. I remember waking up cold one night-a deep, penetrating cold that the blankets couldn't hold back. I climbed out of my bed in the upstairs bedroom of that small farmhouse and padded out into the hallway. The house was silent but for the howl of the wind. I crept to the wooden balcony that overlooked the living room below and peered over the railing.

The sight was surreal, something from a dream. Below, in the glow of a single kerosene lamp, was my foster father. He was shoveling. But he wasn't outside. He was in the middle of the living room, shoveling snow into a large metal tub. Snow depths had been so deep that winter that they covered the heights of the downstairs windows and were heavy enough to cave in the front door of the house. A great, glittering drift had invaded our home, spilling across the braided rug and onto the hardwood floor. Now, in the middle of the night, my foster father was removing the worst that Mother Nature had offered, his breath puffing in the frigid air, each shovelful a soft whump as it landed in the tub. He worked steadily, patiently, as if this were just another farm chore. That image—the quiet man battling the indoor blizzard by lamplight—is seared into me. Not as a trauma, but as a testament. A memory of being safe inside, even when the world was literally breaking in.

I remember several months after I was brought into the Roeters family that they would bring in a new baby. This baby would be their second biological child. Her name was Meaghan. Her arrival was a soft revolution. Suddenly, the attention was no longer solely on me. Now it was on a newborn infant, with a shock of black hair-which would later turn to the brightest blonde-and the helpless, captivating smiles and giggles that came with any newborn child. The house filled with new sounds: the gentle rocking of a cradle, the soft shushing, the sweet, milky scent of her.

In some ways, it was a relief to have the attention taken off of myself. It had been difficult for a long time, having all the focus directed my way. The lack of communication skills and underlying health issues-vague stomach pains, dizzy spells the doctors called "nerves"—had kept me in the center of a concerned circle for months. With Meaghan's arrival, I could retreat to the edges, could observe this new dynamic. I could sit on the floor with Buckey the beaver and just watch this tiny, perfect human, and for a while, the pressure to be understood simply lifted.

Before too much longer, perhaps three or four years, we would move as a family unit to a nearby community of Boyne City, Michigan. The farm was sold; the goat, the chickens, the wide fields, were left behind. It would be here, in Boyne City, a small town nestled between hills and the vast blue of Lake Charlevoix, that I would be enrolled in elementary school. Previously, since I joined the Roeters family, I remember a little red van-nearly the size of a short bus-that would show up to our house in Ellsworth three or four times a week. A kind woman with glasses would work with me at the kitchen table on basic communication skills, on letter sounds, on counting blocks. It was a quiet, one-on-one world.

But the move to Boyne City and starting elementary school for the first time would put me in the presence of peers of my own age. A sea of them. It was at this point in life that we would discover that my lack of communication skills would also affect my ability to properly communicate with people of my own age. The rules were different here. Kids didn't have the patient, deciphering kindness of Mrs. Roeters. They spoke in a rapid, slang-filled code, played games with complex, unspoken rules, and formed alliances I didn't know how to join. My attempts to connect often came out awkward, too loud, or in the wrong context. It was no longer just a problem within my new foster home. It was now an issue everywhere I went.

Between my lack of communication skills and my lack of the common education that a kindergartener would have normally had by that time in their life, I was doomed. I did not properly complete kindergarten but instead had to repeat it—or something similar to it-called Junior Primary. It was a step that the Boyne City Elementary School had, a holding pattern for kids who weren't quite ready, rather than just shoving a student on to first grade. The label "Junior Primary" felt like a brand, a public announcement of my failure to launch.

On a personal standpoint, looking back to my early elementary school days, I recall having difficulty with students that I had thought were either bullies or just mistreated me in general. Faces contorted in laughter I didn't understand, names called that I sensed were insults but couldn't parse, games where I was always "it." But it would turn out later that some of my memories of that period of time were a little spacey, the line between victim and instigator blurred by my own confusion. I had problems getting along with other students, evidently. My foster family would recite throughout my life that I had difficulty getting along with other students and at one point, in a moment of overwhelming frustration, even shoved a girl in a wheelchair off of an auditorium stage. These are not memories that I personally have. My mind has blanked them out, protecting me from the shame of my own actions. But the inability to get along with other students was very pronounced to me throughout the following years growing up. And my memory, in its protective custody, holds very little information of negativity, from my part, within the home. Other than the lack of communication skills and what seemed to be a language of my own, the home remained a sanctuary, even when I was its most chaotic element.

At this point, my foster sibling Scott was no longer living in the home. He had gotten into a large amount of trouble after he stole my foster father's truck. This incident happened back in Ellsworth, a final, dramatic act of rebellion. As a consequence, he was placed elsewhere. Brian was no longer in the home either. He had moved downstate to Mt. Pleasant, chasing a freedom he felt was stifled in our family. He had run into a lot of problems with our foster parents, clashing wills and broken curfews, and had decided on his own to leave.

At this time, this was a profound, unspoken relief to myself and my foster brother Berend. For since shortly after we had left Ellsworth, Brian had, on multiple occasions, done things to Berend and me sexually. They were not acts of violence, but of a terrifying, confusing coercion-whispered threats in shared bedrooms, manipulations in the shadowy barn. These instances caused a lot of fear and a thick, choking frustration between the foster family's older biological son and myself. Frustrations that couldn't be put into words at that time in our lives. We had no vocabulary for the betrayal, the guilt, the shame. They were instances that we individually endured and, unknowingly-for we never spoke of it to each other until we were grown men-shared between ourselves. His departure lifted a silent, suffocating weight from the house.

Our oldest foster sibling, Earlene, was repeatedly in and out of our family, however always in contact. She would never leave our family in the past, and we never forgot her. She would just be part of the family once in a while throughout our entire lives, arriving for holidays or summers, her laughter a familiar, welcome sound. But for the most part, she maintained a life on the reservation in Northern Michigan where she originally originated from, and then later she would follow us out of Michigan when we moved. She was a constant that you could count on. Someone whose love wasn't bound by walls or addresses. Someone who never disappeared from the heart of the family. She will never be forgotten.

In June of 1992, my adoptive mother would once again give birth to another child. With a bright red head full of hair, Pieter brought another wave of joy into the family that we much needed. After the tensions and departures, his arrival was a fresh beginning. He was a squalling, vibrant bundle of new life. Although he had some respiratory-related issues from the time of birth, issues that required an ultraviolet light over his cradle at night, giving his crib a strange, sci-fi glow, those were issues that he would grow out of shortly after. We would all take turns watching him, his tiny fingers curling around ours, a symbol of innocence and forward motion.

For much of this young adolescent period of time in my life, I was still grasping onto trying to communicate properly with people around me. I was now 9 years old. I was 2 years behind everyone else in my grade at school, a fact that hung over me every time

I lined up with the shorter, younger kids. And the basic health issues-originally thought to be just stress-related stomach aches and headaches -slowly progressed into being more deep-seated, mysterious issues that doctors didn't have an answer for. I was poked, scanned, and questioned. My adoptive family would grow frustrated with the lack of answers, the medical bills piling up beside the shrugged shoulders of specialists. And I would grow more frustrated not being understood, failing to know how to communicate the strange, internal weather of my own body to the people around me.

I missed a lot of school at this point in my life. Not just because of the social misunderstandings, but because of repetitive, crippling stomach issues that always had me feeling like something was tearing out of my belly on a daily basis. A sharp, twisting pain that would leave me curled on the bathroom floor. Something that never got better in my younger years, a constant, gnawing companion. Some of my responses to these frustrations-once again with a lack of memory of specific instances-spiraled into a lot of frustration mutually with my adoptive parents. There were slammed doors, nights where I would hide in the closet, their voices outside threaded with worry and exhaustion.

At the age of nine, I had just been finally officially adopted into the family. The court ceremony was brief, a judge smiling down at me. I now had the last name of Roeters officially set in stone. It was supposed to be a finale, a "happily ever after" stamp. However, frustrations continued to build-my pain, their helplessness, the chasm of miscommunication between us-until the point that a family counselor, out of ideas and fearing for the stability of the entire household, recommended that I be placed into what was called Whaley's Children's Center in Flint, Michigan. It was presented as a "therapeutic residential placement," a place where I could get "intensive help."

But for the first time in my life, I felt like I had been abandoned. The drive to Flint felt like a death march. When they left me at the sterile, institutional building, with its locked doors and humming fluorescent lights, a piece of my soul shattered. I felt lost in a way I never had before, even when taken across borders. And for the first time in my life, I felt like I had experienced a loss that had fractured my world. The family I had finally, officially belonged to had driven away, and I was alone with my pain and a room full of strangers who were just as broken as I was.

I wasn't in Whaley's Children's Center for very long. A matter of months, though each day felt like a year. I remember it was just after the beginning of the following year, in 1993, the gray slush of January still on the ground, when my adoptive family came back. They didn't call ahead. They just arrived. Mr. Roeters' beard seemed even redder against the pallid winter light. Mrs. Roeters' eyes were filled with a determined tears. "We made a mistake," was all she said, hugging me so tightly I could hardly breathe. "We're all going together."

Leaving Whaley's Children's Center and headed for our new state of Colorado, I felt a shift deeper than just geography. I would be leaving behind problems that I would not carry with me to our new home-or at least, I vowed I would not carry them in the same way.

Among the health issues that were not understood was the stark, visible fact that I could never grow hair, and that I had worn hearing aids since the time I was four years old. These were not just medical details; they were the bullseyes on my back in the world of children. Prior to being placed into Whaley's, my parents, with the best of intentions, had tried to fit me with a wig-a sandy-brown, synthetic cap meant to hide my bare scalp. They thought it would shield me, keep me out of cruel games like "Monkey in the Middle," where I was always the target. But the wig was an itchy, obvious lie. I finally discarded it myself in a fit of hot shame, or perhaps it was ripped off my head by a mean student during a chaotic recess—the memories blend into one sensation of exposure. Once it was gone, the students' attention simply shifted. They then realized, with fresh malice, the small, flesh-colored devices hooked over my ears. Hearing aids. Devices that stuck out like a sore thumb to young, evil minds, something to flick, to whisper about, to mock the static they sometimes emitted..

In the quiet darkness of the station wagon, watching Michigan's frozen fields give way to the flat, endless expanse of Indiana, I made a silent, firm decision. The wig would never touch my head again. The hearing aids, which felt less like helpers and more like badges of vulnerability, would stay buried at the bottom of my duffel bag. I was done with the props meant to make me look "normal." In the back of my mind, however, I also knew this act of defiance would come at a cost. It would fall back onto my communication skills. Without the aids, the world would grow muffled again; conversations would become guessing games. But the trade-off felt necessary. The clarity wasn't worth the target.

Yet, for all its pain, Whaley's Children's Center had helped me in a raw, unexpected way. It hadn't taken away my anxieties and fears—they were still there, coiled tight in my stomach. But it had shown me my own resilience. In that sterile place, stripped of all familiar comfort, I had learned to watch, to listen with my eyes, to navigate a system. I knew, with a certainty that felt hard-won, that with this move to Colorado, I was not the same terrified, silent boy the Roeters family had first taken in from a porch with a runaway goat.

And when they came for me, it was with an immediate move for the entire family to Craig, Colorado. They had sold the house in Boyne City. They had packed everything. The decision wasn't made from sheer desperation alone; it was also pulled forward by a specific hope. Mr. Roeters had secured a promising job at the hospital in Craig-a chance to return to his professional hospital services as he had in Michigan, work he loved, but on a grander scale, with better pay and a new house... It was an opportunity that felt heaven-sent, a tangible fresh start that offered not just distance from our struggles, but a concrete better future for all of us. For Pieter, whose lungs still sometimes struggled with Michigan's damp, the dry, high-altitude air of Colorado was prescribed as potentially beneficial. For me, it meant a school district none of us had ever been to, where the label "Junior Primary" and the story of the girl in the wheelchair weren't waiting in every teacher's file. The move was an escape, yes, but it was also an embrace-of new air, new land, and a new chance for every single one of us to be seen for who we were becoming, not just for the problems we had been.

A fresh start, for all of us, together. And so, not only was I reunited with my family, we-as an entire family-were moving halfway across the country to a new state, to mountains instead of lakes, to a vast western sky that promised, if not answers, then at least a new kind of air to breathe.

The past, with all its locked doors and indoor snowstorms, its silent traumas and failed communications, was in the rearview mirror. The road ahead was long, and unknown, but for the first time in a long time, I was in the car with them, all of us headed in the same direction.

As I sat in the car on the long drive to Colorado, my mind-quieter now, resolved-drank in the changing world outside the window. We left the forests and the great, gray expanse of the Great Lakes behind, watching the land slowly flatten and stretch out into vast, treeless plains. The sky seemed to grow larger, a huge bowl of endless blue. Then, almost imperceptibly at first, the earth began to rumple and rise in the distance. The flatness gave way to gentle foothills, which then gathered themselves into serious, snow-capped mountains. Everything was different. The very air seemed to change, growing lighter and sharper. And my mindset was different, too. I was observing, not just enduring.

As I sat in the car, while my mother tried to play road games from the front passenger seat in a cheerful, persistent voice-games such as picking out letters of the alphabet from license plates or passing billboards—l quietly looked at my siblings around me instead. My older brother Berend was approximately 14 years old, stretched out and lanky, his face turned toward the window with a thoughtful expression. I was now 10, tucked between bags and blankets. My little sister Meaghan, was approximately five, maybe six, her blonde hair in a messy ponytail, chattering excitedly about every cow and horse she saw. And my youngest brother Pieter was just about two years old, asleep in his car seat, his head lolling, a faint wheeze in his breath that seemed quieter out here. I could see by looking at their faces the pure, uncomplicated joy and awe in their minds as our drive continued west. They saw adventure. I saw a chance to disappear and reappear as someone new.

Along the way, my parents stopped at different landmarks and state parks-the Badlands of South Dakota, a vast, painted desert of striated rock; the looming monument of Devil's Tower in Wyoming, rising from the earth like a giant's tree stump. It was something they had decided would continue as a tradition while we resided in Colorado. "We're not just moving," my dad said, stamping his boots on the gravel at a scenic overlook. "We're explorers now." Everything was surreal. The scale of the landscape made our old problems feel small and far away. This wasn't just a new life for myself; it was a new life for everybody in that car, a shared story we were driving into.

The only anchor to the familiar, the only distraction from the overwhelming newness, was the normalcy of the whiff of cigarette smoke coming from my dad as he drove. The familiar acrid scent mixed with the new smells of dry grass and pine that flooded in through the cracked windows. It was a smell of before, carried into the after.

The drive from Michigan to northwest Colorado- with the sightseeing, the cheap motels with vibrating beds, the picnics at roadside tables-would take approximately four days. Four days in a rolling metal capsule, suspended between a past we were shedding and a future we couldn't yet imagine.

For those four days, we were nowhere and everywhere, a family unit sealed in motion, and for the first time in a very long time, the motion felt like it was moving toward something, and not just away.

When we first moved to Craig, Colorado, our new life began in a modest, pale-yellow house on the north end of School Street. The neighborhood was quiet, with more sagebrush than lawn, and the air held the clean, dusty scent of the high desert. Our home was near the north edge of town, where the paved grids of the community seemed to pause, as if catching their breath before giving way to the vast, open rangeland. A crossroad called Sandrock

Drive lay just a few houses away, a name that promised adventure just by the sound of it.

The people were nice in a straightforward, Western way-a nod from a neighbor, a wave from a passing truck. The house itself was nice, too: small, but filled with new light from windows that framed views of rolling hills instead of dense Michigan forest. It felt like a blank page.

And then, I met Ty St. John. He lived directly across the road, a boy with sun-bleached hair and a grin missing a tooth. He saw me watching from our porch one afternoon, walked right over, and asked if I wanted to see his fort. Just like that. No staring at my head, no side-eyed glance at my ears. I was sensing a new form of freedom-not just from my past, but the profound, simple freedom of having a friend who did not tease me and treat me differently because of my own differences. It was an unearned, miraculous grace. Even though, as with every new friend I would gain over time, Ty would soon realize I had medical problems that left me constantly feeling ill-days where I'd have to lie down in the fort, dizzy and nauseous, or cut a bike ride short with a cramping stomach. But his response wasn't mockery; it was a shrug. "We can just hang out here," he'd say, and that was that.

Between my newfound friend and me, we would together, on battered bicycles with knobby tires, discover the map of our new community. We'd pedal down the empty back streets, past the lumber yard smelling of fresh-cut pine, along the railroad tracks, and out to the edges where the town dissolved into scrub and sky. It seemed, since moving away from Michigan, that my parents had released the restraints off of me. The constant, worried supervision was replaced with a common, trusting note: "Be home before dark."

This was an experience I was not used to-this trust, this assumption of competence. It made me stand a little taller.

Relatively speaking, the city of Craig was not a very large community. To a ten-year-old on a bicycle, however, it was an empire. You could literally ride from the elementary school on the east side to the city park on the Yampa River on the west in less than 45 minutes, the wind in your face, master of your own destiny. And just on the north side of town, past Sandrock Drive, was the landmark that gave the road its name: a set of sprawling, weathered sandstone rocks, honey-colored in the afternoon sun. They gave way to a hundred climbing adventures, hidden crevices, and secret ledges that Ty introduced me to from the very beginning. We'd scramble up the rough, warm rock, our pockets full of stolen cookies, and sit on top, kings of all we surveyed-the quiet town below, the endless expanse of ranches and mountains beyond.

It was a wonderful new life. The sharp, dry air, the boundless sky, the solid warmth of the sandstone under my hands-all of it was a sensory antidote to the damp, closed-in memories of Michigan. At times, perched on those rocks with Ty, the vast western horizon filling my vision, I almost forgot about Michigan entirely. The past wasn't gone, but it was finally, blessedly, out of sight.

As a ten-year-old when we first moved to Craig and into that first home on School Street, I was blissfully unaware that my parents had already been searching for a bigger house for our growing family within the community. The yellow house was just a starting point, a temporary harbor. Before the first chill of winter had firmly begun to bite, we packed again and moved about a mile away, to 890 Finley Lane.

This new house was different-larger, two-storied, with a wide porch and a sprawling backyard. It sat directly across the street from the imposing brick facade of Craig High School, and was much closer to the elementary school where I would be starting third grade. But the move came with a quiet cost: it was now too far to easily see my new friend Ty on a daily basis. The simple, magical run across the road was gone. Him and I would be in the same elementary school, a small consolation, but with the winter months coming on, burying the town in deep, silent snow and brittle cold, it wouldn't be so easy to ride my bicycle to his home until the following spring. A season of friendship, so vivid and new, was suddenly put on hold by geography and weather.

Once we were moved into our new home, however, life quickly filled the space Ty had left. I would quickly find new friends nearby. Eddie Yeash and Howard Bauer lived directly across the street from our home, in identical houses with steep driveways perfect for sledding. They were both in my grade-a fact that offered immediate belonging, even though I was still two years older than everyone else in my class, a lingering, unspoken stigma that would never quite go away. Eddie was skinny as I was and boisterous, Howard quieter with a thoughtful gaze and very tall. They accepted my presence without fanfare. Eddie and Howard would quickly become full-time companions by my side, a trio exploring the alleyways behind Finley Lane, building snow forts in the vacant lot, and trading Garbage Pail Kids cards on the high school steps... we too, as a trio, would explore the sand rocks together that were now across the street from the high school.

Our families grew close. All of our parents would take turns babysitting the others, a rotating system of trust that allowed them to have time alone with their spouses, to steal dinner dates and private time. On those nights, the three of us would rule one of our houses, gorging on popcorn and watching movies on the VCR, a unit of bundled-up, chaotic joy. It was a new kind of normalcy, woven from simple routines and shared custody.

It's kind of funny when I look back at it now, with the clarity of decades. Approximately thirty years after moving into that house, long after our stay in Colorado had ended, I would sit down to write a series of books. Within those books, titled It's In The Blood, I used this exact house-890 Finley Lane-as a setting. I gave its porch, its creaking stairway, and its view of the high school to my characters. And I used the names of many of my friends, including Eddie Yeash, borrowing the solid, real sound of them to anchor fiction in the soil of memory. It was my way of honoring a time and place that had, for a little while, saved me.

As for Ty St. John... sometimes it's weird how friends come and go out of our lives. Regardless of the importance of that relationship—or friendship —sometimes people appear and vanish like figures in a revolving door, leaving a gust of cold air and a memory of warmth in their wake. I don't believe it's really ever intentional. I think it's just the forces of nature-moves, seasons, the slow drift of growing up-pulling people in different directions. Ty was an awesome friend. A true first friend in a new world. It would be cool to be reunited with him sometime in the future, to share a coffee and say, "Remember the sand rocks?"

But we lost contact with each other years ago, as children do. Life carried on. I recently found out, about two years ago while falling down an internet rabbit hole, that his father had passed away. I also learned, with a jolt of pride, that his father had become the mayor of Craig for a number of years. Suddenly now, as I'm writing this, I'm having flashback memories, not just of Ty, but of his parents: his mother's kind smile, his father's firm hand on my shoulder. They had included me on multiple occasions as a child—in t-ball games where I stood confused in the outfield, at backyard barbecues where I felt shy but welcome, in simple family functions that made me feel grafted onto something sturdy and good.

I guess sometimes it's scary, seeing how people come and go out of your life like a revolving door. You catch a glimpse of a face you loved, the door spins, and they're gone, taking a piece of your history with them into the unknown. But they leave behind the imprint of their presence, the shape they made in your life. Ty left me with the taste of freedom and the warmth of sandstone. And that, it turns out, is a thing you can keep forever.

Chapter 4

Life in the new home at 890 Finley Lane settled, after the flurry of the move, into a steady, reliable rhythm. It had become routine. There were daily adventures with my new friends, Eddie and Howard. Our world was the few blocks around Finley Lane-the high school parking lot after hours, the ditch behind Howard's house that became a raging river during spring melt, the 7-Eleven where we pooled change for Slurpees. My brother, Berend, now navigating the social labyrinth of high school across the street, had made his own friends, his life expanding in ways that felt grown-up and distant. My sister, Meaghan, had also become of age for finding friends of her own, her laughter now echoing with other girls' voices from her bedroom upstairs. Our family was putting down roots, each of us branching out in the thin Colorado soil.

My dad's employment at The Memorial Hospital, which had started as a managerial role, had grown over time into something substantial. He became the hospital administrator, a fact noted with quiet pride. He'd leave in a button-down shirt and a tie, carrying a briefcase-a far cry from the flannel and work boots of the Michigan farm. His success offered a new kind of stability. And with that foundation, my mother, alongside Eddie's and Howard's mothers, channeled their formidable energy into a venture of their own. They started a business called 'Rag Time Rugs.' The concept was ingenious and thrifty: they collected old denim jeans, cut them into long, continuous strips, and wove them into heavy, durable rugs on a large, intimidating loom that quickly overtook a large portion of our basement. The constant thunk-thunk-thwack of the loom became the heartbeat of the house, a sound of industry and creation. The air carried the faint, clean smell of denim and machine oil. It was a shared project, a tapestry of friendship and enterprise that mirrored the one us boys were living out above ground.

It was during this period of settled routine and growing stability that both of my parents turned a new, more urgent kind of attention toward my personal health issues. I believe this was promoted by a short, alarming string of multiple minor fractures that I had recently experienced-a constellation of injuries that seemed to defy the normal rough-and-tumble of boyhood. There were a couple of separated ribs from a simple fall off my bike where the handlebar jabbed my side. Teeth too easily knocked out by light impacts that should have only caused a fat lip. A broken toe from stubbing it on the basement stairs. My body seemed strangely fragile, like china wrapped in boy-skin.

Then, as usual, the old issues resurfaced with new, adolescent ferocity. My hearing, long neglected since I'd buried my aids in the duffel bag, had once again become an issue at the forefront. Teachers noted I wasn't responding, that I seemed lost during class discussions. The world was steadily muffling, and my strategy of lip-reading and guessing was failing. And most painfully, especially as I was becoming a teenager, was the absolute inability to grow hair of any kind, anywhere. This wasn't just a childhood oddity anymore; it was a glaring, defining deviation in the hormonally charged world of middle school. It became agonizingly public during required gym class showers-a scene of stark exposure where my smooth scalp and hairless body stood out amidst the fuzz and fledgling mustaches of my peers. The whispers, the stares, the stifled laughs were a silent violence. That scene, repeated and dreaded, eventually caused me to skip gymnasium altogether, forging notes or simply enduring the detentions that followed. It was easier to be punished for disobedience than to be nakedly vulnerable.

The routine of Finley Lane-the friends, the loom's rhythm, my father's steady job-formed the backdrop to a more pressing drama: the mystery of my own body was deepening, and its demands could no longer be ignored or hidden in the vastness of a new state.

I recall that in this time period, my parents' concern shifted into high-gear action. They drove me across the state, to Denver, a couple of times for appointments at the Denver Children's Hospital-a place that seemed both awe-inspiring and terrifying in its sheer scale and sterile competence. These weren't check-ups; they were deep-dive investigations, quests for a root cause. None of these appointments I would ever want to repeat again in my life. They exist in my memory as chambers of polished fluorescence and low, clinical voices, places where I was transformed from a boy into a fascinating, faulty specimen.

Twice, I had spinal taps. The memory is one of profound violation-being curled into a tight ball on a cold table, the sharp, burning sting of local anesthetic, followed by a deep, impossible pressure as a needle sought the fluid around my spine. It was a pain that wasn't just in the back; it resonated through my hips, down my legs, a weird, electric wrongness. I was told not to move, to breathe slowly, while inside I was screaming. The headaches that came afterward were monumental, as if my skull were collapsing inward from the vacuum left behind.

And then there was the other test. A procedure whose official name I've blotted out, but whose sensations are etched in fire. It was some sort of metabolic test that required the removal of nearly every drop of blood from my body, much like dialysis, but without the gentle hum of a machine to distance you from the process. This test was done without anesthesia of any kind. I was awake for the entire, surreal procedure. I lay on a gurney and watched as thick tubes were connected to needles in my arms. I felt my own blood leaving me-a slow, draining weakness, a growing chill that started in my fingertips and crept inward toward my core. A profound lightheadedness took over, and the world faded to a gray, buzzing tunnel. The actual test, they said, took place in that suspended, nearly bloodless state. Then, just as disorientingly, the cooled blood was pushed back into my veins. The return was a violent, burning invasion, as if ice-cold sludge were being forced through every vessel. This particular test was nearly as painful as the spinal taps, but it was a total bodily assault-it affected my entire being, my very sense of self, rather than just focusing on my spine. That procedure and the spinal taps were the absolute worst of my testing, islands of agony in a sea of worry, and they are still deep-seated in my memory, pristine in their horror.

All in the mix of this same desperate, probing time, my body found new ways to betray its fragility. I contracted chicken pox. For most children, it's a rite of passage, itchy and uncomfortable but manageable. For me, it became a crisis. The way my body reacted was extreme -a fever that spiked uncontrollably, lesions that seemed to merge into angry, swollen plains of inflammation. I remember one night in particular, my skin on fire, my breathing becoming shallow and ragged. My father, his face a mask of pure panic, scooped me up from my bed, wrapped me in a blanket, and rushed me out to the car in the middle of the night. The cold Colorado air was a shock against my burning skin. I remember the sting of the frost on the driveway through the blanket, the desperate fumble of keys, the roar of the engine as he sped toward the local hospital in

Craig. He was talking to me, his voice tight with fear, but I was too far gone in the fever, too helpless to respond. My body always overreacted to every little element-viruses, impacts, allergens-that most children endured without incident. It wasn't just sick; it was alarmist. It sounded sirens over skinned knees and turned common childhood illnesses into full-blown emergencies.

These experiences—the terrifying trips to Denver, the traumatic procedures, the midnight dashes to the local ER-painted a stark picture. The stability of Finley Lane, the success of Rag Time Rugs, my father's polished shoes: all of it existed in a parallel universe to the one I inhabited, a world of unpredictable pain and medical mystery that no amount of denim rugs or administrative titles could fix.

Through all the testing, the probing, the hope invested in specialists with diplomas on Denver walls, no definitive diagnosis or cures were ever found. Not until recently did we find the truth... However, in that long and frustrating journey, we began to find ways to resolve some of the specific symptoms that made daily life so difficult. It was detective work of elimination. We learned, for instance, that I was severely lactose intolerant- something that wasn't a common household concept in those days. Cutting out milk and ice cream brought a startling reduction in the crippling stomach cramps. We discovered I was actually allergic to meat items we had not been aware of before, common things like poultry and certain cuts of pork. Once we understood these triggers and stripped them from my diet, the constant, low-grade nausea and many of the mysterious rashes and fevers began to recede.

But fixing symptoms was not the same as fixing the core problem. It did not make my bones stronger or less prone to fracture. It didn't restore my hearing, other than leading me, reluctantly, to obtain new hearing aids -a pair of behind-the-ear models I accepted with a heavy heart, the ghosts of schoolyard taunts whispering in my memory. I was still living with the traumatizing moments from the past that had originally caused me to stop wearing them in the first place. And knowledge of symptoms, however helpful, never prompted a single hair to grow on my scalp or body. The mirror remained a stark reminder of a fundamental difference no diet could change.

What my parents did do, however—in a move of profound and loving wisdom-was to focus on building a life around the mysteries, rather than letting the search consume it. Along with Eddie's parents and Howard's parents, they put all three of us kids into Cub Scouts. It was a collective decision, a commitment to normalcy.

Cub Scouts was an island of pure, structured fun. It gave way to other opportunities: friends from different parts of town, learning experiences through the rituals and requirements of the Cub Scouts of America. I learned to tie knots I'd soon forget, to identify local birds, to carve a block of pine into a crude racing car for the legendary Pinewood Derby. The blue uniform shirt felt like a cloak of belonging. I was just another scout, my differences softened by the shared focus on achievements and patches. Later, we would graduate together into Boy Scouts, Troop 157, trading the blue for tan, moving from the church basement to week-long camping trips in the Flat Tops Wilderness.

For the most part, other than the obvious physical differences I could never shed, Scouting allowed me to live a little bit of a normal life. Sitting around a campfire with Eddie, Howard, and a dozen other boys, the smoke in my eyes, the taste of burnt marshmallow on my tongue, the sound of laughter muffled by my hearing aids-in those moments, I wasn't a medical puzzle. I was a Scout. I was part of a team building a bridge, or hiking a trail, or trying to decipher the Morse code handbook. The focus was outward, on the world and the task at hand. It was a reprieve, and perhaps the closest thing to a cure I would ever get: not for my body, but for my spirit.

Although nothing about my health would ever be perfect, life had undeniably become easier, its edges softened by the knowledge we had painstakingly gathered over time. The days of unexplained, debilitating pain became less frequent. I learned to read my body's warnings, to avoid the foods that were poison to me, to brace myself a little differently in a world that felt physically unforgiving. There was a fragile equilibrium. We held onto a quiet, persistent hope that something in the future—some new test, some brilliant researcher-would at least deliver a name, a diagnosis. Something concrete we could grasp onto for deeper help, a key to the final locked door.

Our stay on Finley Lane, the house of the loom and the high school view, would come to an end in about three years. It was right about my 13th birthday, or shortly after, that the familiar boxes reappeared and we made one more move within the community of Craig. This time, it was to a house on a quiet road called Exmore Place, approximately a mile and a half west of town, where the streets began to thin out and the land opened up toward the high desert plateaus. It felt like moving to the edge of the world, a place of greater silence and bigger skies.

But before making this move—just shortly before-I celebrated my 13th birthday. And with that milestone came eligibility for another program, one that would not replace Cub Scouts or Boy Scouts, but would run powerfully side-by-side with them. This program was through the local Craig Police Department: the Police Explorers.

Just like a Cub Scout or Boy Scout uniform, the Police Explorers came with another uniform altogether-but this one carried a different weight, a different kind of authority. It was a crisp, navy-blue shirt with sharp creases, dark trousers, and a wide leather belt. The uniform included official patches on the shoulders and, most significantly, a badge that indicated I was a Police Explorer. Slipping that shirt on for the first time, I felt a transformation. This wasn't about camping or crafts; this was about order, responsibility, and a tangible connection to the adult world of law and safety.

The program was intensely interesting and unique in its access. It allowed us, starting at the age of 13, to ride along with local police officers while they were on duty. I would sit in the passenger seat of a black-and-white cruiser, a clipboard on my knees, listening to the crackle and hum of the police radio. We were taught how to use it properly, to understand the cryptic 10-codes that painted a picture of the town's nightly life-"10-4" for acknowledgment, "10-20" for location, "10-50" for an accident. We learned the importance of public safety, of observation, of being a calm presence. For a boy whose own body often felt chaotic and unreliable, the structure was intoxicating. Here was a system of clear rules, clear communication, and clear purpose. In the Explorer uniform, my differences seemed to recede behind a shield of sanctioned authority. I wasn't the fragile kid; I was an Explorer, learning to protect and serve. It was another kind of belonging, one forged not around a campfire, but in the charged, purposeful quiet of a patrol car rolling through the sleeping streets of Craig.

In addition to the new uniform and the new role in society, I found a beautiful synergy in my school life. I was coincidentally, in eighth grade, taking a class called 'The Law and You.' It was a class designed to demystify the legal system, to help us understand our rights and responsibilities, and to see how the law touched everyday life. The textbook explanations of probable cause and due process came alive for me because I'd seen their real-world echoes from the passenger seat of a cruiser. There were a few special days, with prior permission, that I would wear my Police Explorers uniform to school specifically for this class. Walking the halls in that uniform on those days was a profound experience. The usual glances directed at my hearing aids or my smooth scalp were momentarily replaced with looks of curiosity, even respect. In that classroom, I wasn't just a student; I was a participant, someone with a foot in both worlds. I could contribute, referencing a ride-along or a 10-code, and for once, my voice carried a different kind of authority.

I would continue with the Police Explorers, thriving in this unique space, for about a year and a half. It became a core part of my identity. Then, in a single, bewildering moment, it was all torn away.

The day it happened started like any other at the department. I was a little bit more excited than usual, buzzing with that youthful energy most kids get—maybe I'd aced a test, maybe I was just happy to be there. I came into the police department, the familiar smell of industrial cleaner and coffee in the air, and immediately saw an officer I genuinely liked and admired, someone I'd ridden with many times. Her name was Officer Peggy. She had a no-nonsense demeanor but a kind smile, and she'd always taken time to explain things. When I saw her that day, my excitement spilled over. I greeted her enthusiastically, engaged in a quick, happy conversation about an upcoming Explorer event. As we finished talking and began to head in opposite directions down the hall —me toward the Explorer ready room, her toward the briefing room-I turned around, reached out, and gave her a friendly, pat on the back. It was the same kind of jovial, physical gesture I'd seen other people do, a "see you later" punctuation. "Catch you later, Peggy!" I said, my smile wide and guileless.

The reaction was not what I expected. She stiffened. The friendly light in her eyes vanished, replaced by a flat, professional opacity. She didn't say anything to me then. But later that afternoon, I was summoned to the Explorer advisor's office. I was informed, in cold, formal terms, that my action had been reported as inappropriate physical contact. The word "assault" was used. I was stunned, a cold numbness spreading from my core. I tried to explain, to convey the complete lack of malice, the simple, friendly intent. But the system I had so revered had no room for my confused, adolescent context. The verdict was absolute. I was terminated from the Police Explorers program effective immediately. I was to turn in my uniform, my badge, my clipboard.

The trauma of that expulsion was deep and lasting. wasn't just about losing the activities or the rides. It was the violent contradiction. The program that had taught me about intent, context, and public service had, in my view, utterly failed to apply those principles to me. I was traumatized by the department's severe response to a moment of playfulness that had held absolutely no intention of harm. The badge that had made me feel seen and valued now felt like a brand of shame. The uniform I had worn with pride was now a costume I had been deemed unworthy to wear. It was a brutal lesson: that the structures I found solace in could also be unforgiving, and that my difficulty reading social cues- a part of my deeper, undiagnosed condition-could have consequences far beyond a social hiccup. The door to that world slammed shut, and the lock turned from the other side.

The door to that world slammed shut, and the lock turned from the other side. In the wake of that expulsion, the ground beneath me felt less certain. But life, in its relentless way, kept bringing new people to my doorstep —sometimes literally.

It was about this time that my older foster sister, Earlene, along with her two children, Warren and Joshua, would make their own momentous move from Michigan to Craig, Colorado. They had been living on the reservation just outside of Escanaba, Michigan, a world of dense forests and the vast, moody expanse of Lake Michigan. Trading that for the high desert plains and mountain vistas of Colorado was a leap across worlds. This move would be just as much of a monumental change for them as it had been for our family almost five years before. When their beat-up station wagon, laden with boxes and toys, pulled into the gravel driveway on Exmore Place, it felt like a piece of my old, fragmented world had miraculously tracked me down and decided to stay.

Joshua was the oldest, a serious-eyed boy of about five with a quiet watchfulness. Warren, between three and four, was a whirlwind of energy and giggles. Their presence immediately changed the energy of our home, filling it with the joyful chaos of toddlerhood.

But for me, the greatest gift was Earlene herself. Her arrival was a balm. Earlene was not just a sister to me; she was a sibling I saw as a sanctuary, a place of unconditional refuge and protection. For most of my life, during her visits, she had been the one who spent hours just sitting with me, hugging me when words failed, holding me through stomach aches and silent frustrations. We had spent countless afternoons engaged in rambling conversations that made me feel we were more like chosen friends than siblings bound by circumstance. Her return felt like a safety net had been reinstated beneath the tightrope I was walking.

I needed that refuge more than ever, because at this point in my life, my relationship with my brother Berend had grown strained and difficult. We were both teenagers now-me in my mid-teens, him in his late teens-and the chasm between our experiences seemed to widen daily. Where once we had shared a silent, painful bond over what Brian had done to us, now we clashed. Berend's frustrations seemed to manifest as a simmering aggression, often directed at me. I believe some of those differences-my health issues, my social struggles, the sheer weight of our individual pasts-caused us to grate against each other in the confined space of adolescence. Earlene's calm, grounding presence became a necessary buffer in our home.

Now that we were living on Exmore Road, in the suburb of Craig called Ridgeview, my social world once again reconfigured itself. I had new friends. And just as had been with Ty after the move from Michigan, I never formally ended my friendship with Eddie and Howard- life simply pulled us in different directions, our orbits altering with the move across town. It was another quiet example of that revolving door of friendship, a process that is sometimes heartbreaking in its passive inevitability. Still, to this day, I carry those awesome, sun-drenched memories of each of my best friends like treasured artifacts, each one a chapter in the story of my becoming.

My new friends-Nathan, Brian, and Steve-all lived nearby within the Ridgeview area. Brian and Nathan were actually brothers. They lived at the top of the road that connected to ours, in a house that always smelled of baked goods and pine sap. They also went to the same small church as we did, which added another layer of shared context. Steve, on the other hand, lived only two houses away from me. His proximity made him a constant.

Steve was about two and a half years older than me and was already navigating the social complexities of high school. This gave him an air of worldly knowledge I found fascinating. Brian was a few years younger and in a lower grade than me, and Nathan was even a year or two younger than Brian himself. Ours was a friendship not of peers, but of proximity and need. But regardless of the age differences, I deeply enjoyed my time with each of them. With Nathan and Brian, it was bikes and board games, explorations in the scrubland behind our houses. With Steve, it was something else—it was an apprenticeship in being older.

Steve, with his high-school mentality and his access to a driver's license, would end up being the person in my life who introduced me to things I perhaps regret today: cigarettes, stolen sips of his father's whiskey, the heady, rebellious talk that felt like a shortcut to adulthood. I remember the first harsh, dizzying drag of a cigarette behind his garage, my body already so alien to me reacting with a cough that felt like it came from my toes. I remember the burn of cheap alcohol, a sensation so violently unpleasant I couldn't understand the appeal, but I pretended I did because Steve did. He wasn't a corrupting force out of malice; he was a teenager testing boundaries, and he simply allowed me to tag along. I still believe he was, in his way, a very good friend. He treated me like I was capable of keeping up, never coddling me for my hearing aids or my hairless head. In his world, I was just the kid from two doors down, ready to be shown the ropes, for better or worse. It was another form of acceptance, however fraught, and in the lonely landscape of my mid-teens, I was grateful for it.

Outside of Boy Scouts, which remained a steady, grounding constant in my life-a world of clear ranks and campfire camaraderie that contrasted sharply with the confusing social codes of high school—my mother worked diligently to cultivate other parts of me. Outside of my friendships with Nathan, Brian, and Steve, she had gotten me enrolled in art classes and piano lessons.

The art classes, held in a sunlit community center room that smelled of turpentine and clay, were a quiet revelation. Here, my difficulty with verbal communication didn't matter. I could speak through pencil shading and watercolor washes. I could lose myself in the texture of charcoal on paper, creating landscapes that mirrored the vast ones outside my window. It was a peaceful, productive solitude.

Piano lessons, however, weren't really my thing. The rigid discipline of scales and the precise notation felt like another language I was expected to master by rote. My heart was already with wind instruments, with the breathy, expressive voice of the saxophone I played in the school band. There was something about the physicality of it-the vibration against my hands, the control of my own breath to create a sound-that felt more authentic to me. But my mother had a habit, born of love and a desire to give us every opportunity, of injecting her ideas of proper hobbies into each one of us kids. Some of it we rebelled from outright. Other times, like with the piano, we just caved in because the effort of resistance was greater than the hour of weekly practice, and because it made her happy to hear the halting notes of "Für Elise" echoing from the living room. It was a small price to pay for the light in her eyes.

Around this time, my sister Earlene and her kids achieved a milestone: they got an apartment of their own. It was a nice, ground-floor unit in the Ridgeview Apartments, located right there in our same quiet neighborhood. The move created more physical and emotional space within our often-tense home on Exmore Road. And for me, it granted longer, more purposeful bike adventures. I would pedal the mile and a half to her place, the dry Colorado wind in my face, to spend afternoons sprawled on her floor with Warren and Joshua, or just talking with Earlene over a cup of tea. Her apartment was a sanctuary-a place without history, without clashes, filled only with the gentle chaos of her little family and her unwavering, calm love.

What I did not realize then was that this arrangement was a quiet preamble to a much larger change. My sister's move out of our house, and my proven ability to navigate myself to her place, would soon turn into a trial run for independence. My parents were planning to make another move, once again prompted by my father's employment. An opportunity had arisen for him back in the Midwest, a step up that couldn't be refused. Their plan, carefully laid, was for me to stay behind in Craig. I would live with Earlene for my final year of high school, providing stability and continuity in my education.

I was, in many ways, looking forward to living with my sister. The idea of a home led by her calm presence, free from the escalating tensions with Berend, felt like a relief. However, at the time, I wasn't fully calculating the deeper cost. I was doomed to once again walk away from all my current friends—from Steve's risky tutorials, from Brian and Nathan's brotherly companionship, from the familiar streets of Ridgeview. The revolving door was turning again, but this time, I held the schedule in my hand. I knew the approximate date and time it would swing shut behind me: June, 1988. That knowledge gave the remaining months a poignant, golden-hour glow. Every bike ride, every Scout meeting, every lazy afternoon in the sagebrush took on the soft focus of something cherished and fleeting. I was learning, in a way I hadn't with Ty or Eddie and Howard, to say a conscious, preemptive goodbye.

Living with my sister for those final six months before catching up with my parents was a time of my life I will never forget. I say that now with the heavy weight of hindsight, knowing that years later, I would outlive my sister and both of her children. The sanctuary of that Ridgeview apartment is now a memory-box sealed with grief. Earlene passed away as a result of cirrhosis of the liver, a slow and cruel ending for someone whose spirit was so gentle. Before her, her younger son, Warren- that whirlwind of energy-was accidentally struck by a vehicle late at night while walking along a road wearing dark clothes. The vibrant little boy was gone in a moment of terrible, random chance. And then, more recently, my nephew Joshua, the serious-eyed watcher, also tragically passed away. A large part of my living, breathing memories of my sister and her two beautiful boys now resides eternally within the walls of those modest Ridgeview apartments, a sacred space forever frozen in the Colorado sun of 1988.

When June of 1988 finally rolled around, the goodbye was no longer abstract. I packed my duffel bag once more, said a tight-throated farewell to Earlene, Warren, and Joshua, and boarded a Greyhound bus. My move to catch up to my parents would lead me not to the Midwest, but to Golden, Colorado-a suburb of Denver pressed up against the foothills of the Rockies. It was a world away from Craig. Our new house was situated just east of the entrance to the long Eisenhower Tunnel, that engineering marvel that bores through the continental divide, and within just a few blocks of the Coors Brewery plant, whose malty scent would come to define the air in our neighborhood.

As usual, it was my father's employment that had once again prompted this family move-a promotion that brought us closer to the corporate heart of things. By the time I arrived at the small, beige ranch house on a busy through-street, my brothers and my sister Meaghan were already settled. They had been there for about six months, forging their own paths in this new, crowded ecosystem. I was the last piece slotted into the puzzle, and the picture felt unfamiliar.

Stepping off the bus into Golden was a sensory assault. I wasn't used to the idea of heavy traffic-a constant, roaring river of metal just steps from the front yard. In Craig, the loudest night sound might be a distant coyote or the wind in the sage. Here, it was the hiss of tires on asphalt and the Doppler-effect wail of sirens, day and night. And I wasn't used to such a large, dense population of people. Faces streamed past on sidewalks; voices overlapped in a cacophony at the shopping center; anonymity replaced the familiar, knowing nods of a small town. Both of these entities-the relentless traffic and the tide of strangers-felt more like an intrusion in my life than the comfort of a small rural community. The vast, open sky of Craig felt like it had been traded for a narrower strip of blue, framed by looming foothills and crisscrossed by telephone wires.

The freedom of a bicycle on a dirt road was gone, replaced by bus schedules and curbs. The silence I had cherished was now a commodity I had to seek out behind closed windows. I was a country boy in a suburban grid, and the map I had spent years drawing in my mind- of sand rocks and quiet lanes-was suddenly, utterly obsolete.

Although I had deeply doubted it would ever happen in this loud, anonymous place, a small miracle occurred shortly after my arrival in Golden. I made a friend with a boy who lived nearby. In the sprawl of identical houses and busy lives, a connection sparked. My new friend's name was Adrian Wells. He was approximately two to three years younger than me and physically smaller. Given that I was relatively small for my own age-a lingering effect of the health struggles that had stunted my growth-onlookers who didn't know us would have gotten our ages completely backwards if they had to describe us. We looked like peers, even though I was edging into young adulthood and he was still clinging to the tail end of childhood.

Adrian was about eleven or twelve years old, with a thoughtful demeanor and a surprising passion: he loved camping in a tent in his own front yard. It was a quirky, charming holdover from a more adventurous spirit, perhaps a small rebellion against the suburbia that surrounded him. There were a couple of occasions, treasured breaks from the loneliness of that first summer, when I would participate with Adrian in camping out in that yard. We'd pitch his green nylon dome tent on the crisp lawn, just feet from his parents' lighted windows, and pretend we were in the wilderness. We'd lie in our sleeping bags, talking about school, about comics, about nothing of consequence, the sound of the distant highway a poor substitute for crickets. His house was only about two to three blocks away from mine, a short walk that felt like a journey across a frontier

The only real danger was the gauntlet I had to cross to get there: the extremely busy, four-lane artery of Yampa Avenue that ran directly in front of my house. Crossing it required a sprint and a prayer, a tense calculation of speed and distance that made every visit feel earned. Later, when the summer ended and I began the eighth grade at Everett Junior High, I would have to walk this same path past Adrian's house each morning. Yampa Avenue became my daily trial, a roaring river of metal I had to ford on foot, my heart in my throat as diesel fumes washed over me.

But the traffic was only the first dread. Everett Junior High was the second, and far greater, source of anxiety. It was a massive, brick institution that seemed designed to process students, not to educate individuals. Here, my disabilities-which had been known quantities, however challenging, in the smaller, familiar system of Craig- seemed to baffle and frustrate. My hearing loss, without the consistent use of aids I still resisted, meant I missed instructions and announcements, appearing defiant or distracted. My lack of hair drew stares and whispers in the crowded, merciless hallways. The health issues that necessitated sudden bathroom breaks or days home sick were met with skepticism, not sympathy.

The students weren't very understanding either. The social codes here were more complex, the cliques more rigid. I was an outsider twice over: the new kid, and the different kid. The gentle, if sometimes awkward, acceptance I'd found with friends like Adrian in his yard did not extend into the fluorescent-lit corridors of Everett. In Craig, my differences were woven into the fabric of a small community; here, they were glaring anomalies under a microscope. Some teachers tried, but their understanding was often procedural, not personal -accommodations noted on a form, not a genuine effort to connect. I felt like a problem to be managed, not a person to be taught. The map was not just obsolete here; it was declared invalid. I was lost all over again, this time without the wide, open sky to remind me I could breathe. In the midst of that loneliness, a gift arrived from the past, a bridge thrown across time and distance.

Much to my surprise and soaring joy, my parents had quietly arranged for my old friend Eddie Yeager to visit us in Golden. They had contacted his family, coordinated a weekend, and kept it a secret until his familiar face appeared at our door. I was electrified. I had believed, in the way teenagers do, that I had lost him forever-that he was another casualty of that revolving door, a cherished memory sealed in the amber of Craig. His presence in our beige suburban living room was a living, breathing contradiction to that fear.

Within that reunion, the years and miles melted away. We spent several hours just playing and reminiscing, the two of us sprawled on the shag carpet. We talked about Howard, about BB gun wars in the Finley Lane backyard, shooting at little green army men until they were pocked with dimples. Eddie reminded me of the time his dad had taken us rabbit hunting in the scrubland outside Craig, the cold morning air sharp in our lungs, the profound silence of the hunt. We laughed about the hours we'd spent scrambling up the sand rocks, just as I had with Ty years before, claiming the same ledges and vistas. The visit only lasted one day, a fleeting twenty-four hours, but its impact was permanent. It showed me, with concrete proof, that not all friends disappear forever. Some bonds could stretch across states and re-knit themselves in an instant. It was a lesson in the durability of true connection, a lifeline thrown to me in a sea of change.

Bolstered by that visit, my new friendship with Adrian there in Golden grew stronger and deeper. He became my daily refuge. I would often go over to his house after school and on weekends-any moment I could steal to get away from the busy tension of our own home and to try to put everything behind me: the bafflement of school, the constant rumble of traffic, the feeling of being an alien in this crazy, busy town. Adrian's house was a sanctuary of normalcy. We'd play Nintendo in his basement, the electronic blips and music a universal language. We'd pore over his comic book collection, or just sit in the tent in his yard, talking as the suburban dusk settled around us. In his company, I didn't have to explain myself. I could just be.

Then, in December of 1988, this fragile, hard-won phase of our lives came to a sudden, shocking end. Once again, my father was relocating for a new job. I had known a move was possible—it was the pattern of our lives-but I'd braced for another shift within Colorado, or maybe back to Michigan. The reality was far more vast, and far more remote.

I didn't grasp the enormity until Adrian's father made it real for me. One afternoon, as I was saying a casual goodbye, Mr. Wells stopped me. He had a solemn, kind look on his face. "Come here for a second," he said, and led me into their den. He pulled down a large, colorful globe from a shelf, its axis squeaking. He spun it, his finger finding Golden, a tiny dot in Colorado. Then, slowly, he traced his finger north-up through Wyoming, Montana, across the vast sprawl of Canada-farther and farther, across immense, unmarked wilderness, over the curved top of the world.

His finger didn't stop at the familiar shape of Alaska's panhandle. It kept going, moving northwest across the blank white expanse of the state, past Anchorage, past Fairbanks, out to a lonely nub of land jutting into the freezing waters of the Kotzebue Sound, on the shores of the Chukchi Sea. He tapped it.

"This," he said softly, "is where you're going. Kotzebue, Alaska."

I stared. The name meant nothing to me, but the distance on that curved surface was astronomical. It wasn't a move; it was a voyage to the edge of the habitable world. Golden, Colorado, suddenly looked like the center of civilization. The globe made the abstraction terrifyingly concrete. The sand rocks, Finley Lane, the Ridgeview apartments, even this busy street in Golden-all of it was about to be reduced to a series of points on a line stretching into a remote, frozen landscape I could barely conceive of.

"It's above the Arctic Circle," Mr. Wells added, his voice a mix of awe and sympathy. "Land of the midnight sun. And in winter... polar night."

My breath caught. The words "Arctic Circle" and "polar night" echoed in my head, concepts from geography class suddenly becoming my future. The revolving door wasn't just turning; it was blowing off its hinges, ready to hurl me into a place of eternal summer light and endless winter dark. The sanctuary of Adrian's basement, the warmth of his tent, the very idea of a "neighborhood"-all of it was about to be replaced by a reality I could not yet imagine.

The sanctuary of Adrian's basement, the warmth of his tent, the very idea of a "neighborhood"-all of it was about to be replaced by a reality I could not yet imagine. The oddness of this move, compared to all our past relocations, began to show itself in different, subtle ways almost immediately.

It was evident even in the mundane task of transferring my school records from Everett Junior High. Walking those fluorescent-lit hallways one last time, I stopped by each teacher's classroom. The conversations were unlike any I'd had with them before. When I said I was leaving, their eyebrows shot up. When I said, "Alaska," their expressions shifted to something between disbelief and fascination. Each teacher had some sort of short, animated conversation with me about Northern Alaska -asking about the temperature, the daylight, the wildlife. There was a palpable excitement in their voices. Unfortunately, it was not the excitement of welcoming a new student, nor even the professional concern they might have shown for my struggles earlier in the term. It was the thrill of the exotic, as if I were no longer a student but an adventurer, a character in a story they'd only read about. It was an awkward day, filled with these stilted, surreal exchanges. Students who'd barely glanced at me now stared with open curiosity. Yet, in a strange way, it left my mind with a little ease. The school that had felt so hostile and impersonal was now framing my departure as something extraordinary. It placed a faint, positive note in the back of my mind as I walked out its doors for the last time-not as a failure escaping, but as a traveler embarking.

At home, the physical process of preparing for this move was utterly different from anything we'd done before. In the past, a move meant a frantic weekend of heaving furniture into a rented U-Haul or cramming possessions into the back of our station wagon. It was chaotic, sweaty, and immediate. This time, it was a methodical, almost clinical dissection of our lives. We placed individual items-based on what room of the house they came from-into identical, sturdy cardboard boxes. Each box was numbered with thick black marker. Corresponding numbers were carefully written on a master inventory list, indicating not just the box's contents, but the exact room in a house we'd never seen in Kotzebue where those boxes would go. It felt less like packing and more like cataloguing evidence of a life we were leaving behind, preparing it for storage in a future that was still a blank page. This meticulous process took about a week. The house echoed with the rustle of packing paper and the scratch of marker on cardboard, a slow-motion unraveling.

My friend Adrian came over during those final days and helped me with some of my personal stuff-my books, my model kits, the small treasures of a teenage boy. His presence was a quiet comfort amidst the growing emptiness of my room. In the process, I began to set aside things to give to him: a particularly cool die-cast car, a stack of my favorite comics, a poster. They were tokens, something for him to remember me by. Because of the age difference, and the sheer, insane distance of Alaska, I was painfully aware that these afternoons might be the very last time I ever saw or heard from Adrian. The revolving door was about to spin with such force that reconnection felt mathematically impossible. This was a grim, cold feeling in the back of my mind, a quiet grief I didn't know how to voice. But based on the relentless lessons of the past—with Ty, with Eddie and Howard, with so many others—I had already begun, as a form of self-preservation, to set my mind in the direction of reality. I hugged him goodbye not with a "see you later," but with a "take care of yourself." It was the goodbye of someone who had learned that some doors, once closed, open onto entirely different worlds.

It was about the second week of December in 1988 when our migration to Northern Alaska truly began. The process felt more like deploying on a mission than moving to a new home. It started with us spending a final night at a generic airport hotel in Denver, the kind with thin walls and humming ice machines. Our worldly possessions were already somewhere in the cargo system, just numbers on a manifest. The next morning, in the pitch dark of a winter dawn, we rushed through the chill to Denver's Stapleton Airport, a nervous, sleep-deprived unit about to be launched into the unknown.

The journey unfolded as a series of disconnected, liminal spaces. Between different flights on a massive Boeing 747, we wound up in Seattle, Washington, with its gray, damp skies, and then, several hours later, touched down in Anchorage. The scale of the travel was already sinking in. But then, an error-a snag in the grand plan. I believe it was a weather-related delay, a common antagonist in Alaskan travel. This triggered an unexpected two-night stay at the Hilton hotel in Anchorage. We were stranded, but we had arrived in Alaska, if not our final destination.

Even though we had not yet made it to Kotzebue, the differences I would soon be living with were starting to announce themselves with startling clarity. The Anchorage airport and the Hilton lobby were not decorated with potted plants or abstract art. They were galleries of the north. The walls were dominated by state-record taxidermied animals: a polar bear standing on its hind legs, its mouth a silent roar; a moose with a rack so wide it seemed to frame a doorway; a grizzly caught in a perpetual, powerful stride. These animals were not just large; they were enormous, monstrous in a way that no zoo encounter could convey. And this was only the taxidermied professional job after an animal had passed away. The living versions, I realized with a shiver, were out there, in the dark beyond the runway lights.

Eventually, we boarded a smaller airliner for the final leg. Our next stop was Nome, Alaska. The plane descended through thick clouds, and we never even got off—it was just a layover, a pause to refuel and exchange passengers. But peering out the frost-rimed window during that stop, I was struck by the profound darkness. I looked at my watch: it was only about 3:00 in the afternoon. But outside the windows of the airliner, the world was plunged into a deep, impenetrable blackness, as if it were 3:00 in the morning.

This was my first real experience of the Arctic winter day-or lack thereof. The sun, for all intents and purposes, had abandoned this place.

Within a couple of hours, the engines whined back to life, and we lifted off again into the night. Finally, the captain announced our descent into Kotzebue. The landing was a bumpy affair on a runway carved out of the frozen tundra. And then came the moment that cemented the sheer alien nature of this new life: unlike any other airport I'd ever seen, we didn't taxi to a glowing terminal. The 737 rolled to a stop out on the open tarmac, under the stark, icy glare of floodlights. The doors opened, and a wave of air so cold it felt solid and sharp rushed into the cabin. It was a physical blow. We were instructed to disembark right there, down mobile stairs onto the frozen ground.

This was profoundly weird to me. I'd never seen or heard of such a thing. We were met at the foot of the stairs by a small group-co-workers of my father's from the local hospital, bundled in enormous parkas with fur-rimmed hoods, their breath pluming in thick clouds. The greetings were quick, practical; pleasantries froze in the air. Stepping out of the aircraft and into temperatures that were approximately 30 below zero, I recall a moment of surreal disorientation. I looked at the idling vehicle, a heavy-duty Suburban, and then back at the 737. They were nearly nose-to-nose, like a car meeting a spacecraft on some desolate moon. The sight was something I had never even imagined, something that belonged in a television movie about the Arctic, not in my own life. This was not Colorado. This was not even Earth as I knew it. This was the edge, and we had just stepped off.

Chapter 5

Stepping off that plane was not just an end to the known past; it was the beginning of a future that would form and shape my entire life. The cold that hit me on that tarmac was not merely weather-it was an element, a presence, a force that demanded respect. And the darkness that enveloped us was not simply night; it was a season, a condition of existence that would redefine my understanding of time itself.

The duplex we moved into, owned by the PHS hospital service where my father worked, sat on the frozen ground like a shelter on the moon. Within just a couple days of arriving, we experienced something that cemented the surreal nature of our new home. In the middle of the night-though night and day had lost all meaning in the perpetual dark-we were jolted awake by a sound that seemed impossible: a heavy, scraping, thumping commotion on our roof. It literally sounded like Santa's sleigh landing, reindeer hooves and all. My heart hammered. We all scrambled out of bed, threw on coats over our pajamas, and rushed outside into the bitter cold.

What we found was both absurd and wonderful. Children -neighborhood kids, Inuit children-were sledding off the edge of our roof. The winter snowdrifts, sculpted by relentless Arctic winds, had piled so high against one entire side of our duplex that they formed a smooth, sloping ramp from the ground all the way up to the roofline. The kids had climbed up, launched themselves off the peak, and slid down the drift on plastic sleds, their laughter cutting through the frigid air. It was about 2:00 in the morning, mid-December, and these children were playing in the dark as if it were a summer afternoon. I knew in my mind, even in my sleep-deprived confusion, that this wasn't a matter of disrespect. It was a difference in culture-a world where boundaries were fewer, where the environment was not a barrier but a playground, where the concept of "appropriate hours" bent to the reality of endless night. Our parents, after the initial shock, seemed to understand this too. They shooed the kids off with smiles, not anger. We were the newcomers here. We were the ones who had to learn.

Our first weeks in the new community were not met with the familiar cycle of day and night. At that time of year, Kotzebue was locked in a consistent 24-hour darkness—a deep, velvety twilight that never lifted. The sun, we would come to understand, had abandoned us for a season. We wouldn't witness our first sunrise until about the first week of February, a date we marked on the calendar with anticipation. The weather was brutal in ways I'd never conceived: wind chills that made exposed skin burn and freeze in minutes, the constant creak and groan of the house settling in the cold, the need to plug in the car's engine block heater every night just so it might start in the morning. But no matter how brutal the weather was-in that moment locked in the world of darkness, or months later in the summertime when we would be locked in total daylight, the sun circling the sky without ever setting-we would discover that our new world was absolutely beautiful in every aspect. The darkness held stars so bright they seemed within reach, and the northern lights danced across the sky like living curtains of green and violet. The summer light painted the tundra in impossible shades of gold and amber. It was harsh, but it was magnificent.

We had landed in mid-December. It was only a couple days later that my siblings and I were enrolled in our new schooling systems. Even this most basic of activities -registering for school-revealed differences you would never see in the lower forty-eight states. I was being enrolled into the Kotzebue Middle/ High School, a modern building that rose from the tundra like an outpost of civilization. But the students arriving there told a different story. They came to school on their own snowmobiles, tiny figures buzzing across the white expanse. A few were dropped off by their parents, also on snowmobiles, the machines idling as goodbyes were shouted over the roar. And once in a while, you would witness something that stopped you in your tracks: a student arriving on a dog sled, the team of huskies panting steam into the frigid air, the parent bundled in furs and speaking soft commands in Inupiaq. Though this was a rarity-a beautiful, living connection to a traditional past-it was something you would see once in a while, and it never failed to remind me how far I was from Craig, Colorado.

I remember the faces of the students in that school. They were much different from any classroom I'd ever sat in. For the first time in my life, I was in a school where being a white person made you a minority. Approximately ninety percent of the population of the community- and that school-was Inupiat Eskimo, the indigenous people of the NANA region of Alaska. They were the original inhabitants of this land, with features shaped by millennia of Arctic life: dark, intelligent eyes that crinkled at the corners when they smiled, high cheekbones, hair black as ravens' wings.

Although it felt profoundly weird, even disorienting, to suddenly be part of a minority group after a lifetime of blending into the majority, I was surprised-and deeply moved-by how well I was welcomed. The students, the teachers, the community at large opened their arms to me and the rest of my family. There was no resentment, no cold shoulder. They seemed genuinely curious about us, and genuinely kind. It was my first real lesson in what it felt like to be the outsider, and how grace from the inside can make all the difference.

School lessons were different here, too. You had your basic math, English, and social studies-the standard curriculum of any American school. But then you also had mandatory classes that were utterly foreign to me: Inupiat class, which taught the traditional ways and the ancient language of the people. And there were "Inupiat Days," where the entire school would go out on snowmobiles-sometimes even dog sleds-to learn and understand the traditional ways of living in the Arctic firsthand. These were not field trips in the sense I knew; they were survival training, cultural preservation, living history. Often, these days included topics that could save your life if you were ever to become stranded on the Arctic tundra, winter or summer: how to build a snow shelter, how to read the wind, how to find water, how to respect the land that could kill you if you didn't.

Learning the language was not just an academic exercise; it was the basics of communicating with people in general. Although most people within the school system had the ability to speak English, several of those students' parents or grandparents knew very little English-or sometimes none at all. The elders, the knowledge-keepers, spoke in the old tongue. So learning Inupiaq was vital to learning from them, to understanding the stories and wisdom carried in that language for thousands of years. Sitting in that class, struggling to form guttural sounds my mouth had never made, I realized I was not just attending school. I was being initiated into a culture, a place, a way of being that had endured on this frozen coast since time immemorial. And somehow, impossibly, they were letting me in.

As I'm writing this now, decades later, I'm still trying to find the words within my mind and soul to correctly and accurately represent the differences between living in Colorado and Michigan in the past and moving to Kotzebue. The best phrase that comes to mind— the one that rises from my memory like ice bubbling to the surface of a lead in the frozen sea-is this: it was like moving to another planet. A planet that would hypothetically carry on in the English language, with all the familiar words for homework and dinner and "how was your day," but that was simultaneously overlaid with a traditional native side to it, a parallel dimension that was utterly vital to the area. English was the language of the classroom, of commerce, of the outside world. But Inupiaq was the language of the land itself, of survival, of the elders who knew how to read the sky and the ice in ways that no textbook could teach.

Obviously, when you live within the Arctic Circle, weather is the number one difference-the omnipresent, defining force of existence. Everything else orbits around it. Looking back at my mid-teens, I recall that the weather variances and temperatures, during the winter months, could swing wildly from 32 degrees above zero-without wind chill, a veritable heat wave that would have us peeling off layers-to 128 degrees below zero with the wind chill, a cold so profound that exposed skin would freeze in under a minute, that breath froze in your beard, that the air itself seemed to crystallize and creak.

And I recall, with absolute clarity, that the wind was the major factor in everything. It was not an afterthought; it was the primary character in the daily drama of survival. My adoptive father, Berend Sr., weighed well over 250 pounds-a solid, substantial man who had worked ranches and farms his entire life. I remember watching him one bitter winter day, stepping out of our front door, his boot catching on a drift or a hidden snowbank. Before he could even react, the wind—a sustained, howling force screaming off the Chukchi Sea-caught him. I watched, frozen in disbelief, as it literally blew him across a section of our yard. He tumbled and skidded across the crusted snow, a 250-pound man rolling like a tumbleweed, traveling at least ten to fifteen feet before he was able to dig in his heels, stop himself, and struggle back up to his feet, gasping and laughing at the sheer absurdity of it. If the wind could do that to him, I thought, what could it do to me?

The answer to that question was built into the infrastructure of the community itself. The Kotzebue Elementary School had a fence approximately fifteen to twenty feet tall erected around its entire perimeter. Not around the middle and high school, where we older students were deemed capable of handling ourselves, but only around the elementary school. This fence was not for keeping strangers out or children in, in the usual sense. It was literally in place to prevent the youngest children from being blown off the playground-the same playground that every elementary school has, with its swings and slides and monkey bars, now ringed by a towering barrier that spoke to the raw power of the place. It was a fence against the wind itself.

To understand why the wind held such sway, you have to understand where Kotzebue sits. The community is like an oasis-a fragile spit of land caught between the Bering Strait and the Kotzebue Sound that surrounds it on all perimeter sides. The entire community is essentially a peninsula, a narrow finger of gravel and tundra stretching out toward the Bering Strait, pointing in the general direction of Russia, visible only as a distant, mythical line on the horizon. There are no trees here. No rolling hills. No mountains to break the flow of air. Nothing but flat, open tundra and the frozen sea. The landscape offers no windbreak whatsoever. And so the wind comes through the community every winter at full blast, unimpeded, relentless, a living thing with a voice that howls and

shrieks and moans for days on end.

There have been incidences in the past-and some that I would witness in my own near future-where children and sometimes adults were literally blown off this spit of land and onto the frozen ice that surrounds the community during the winter months. The ice pack, which extends for miles out to sea, is not a safe place to be caught unprepared. Most of these people, thank God, would be found-by search parties on snowmobiles, by the keen eyes of community members who knew the patterns of the drifts. But some were not. Some were taken by the wind and the white, lost to the immense, indifferent beauty of the Arctic. It was a fact of life here, spoken of in hushed tones, a reminder that this planet we had moved to, for all its wonder, was also capable of erasing you without a second thought.

But the weather wasn't the only threat. In the land of the Arctic, you also have four-legged animals that treat the community like it's merely an obstacle in their territory- because, to them, it is. It wasn't unusual for a stray polar bear to stride directly into Kotzebue, wandering down the snow-packed streets as if they were game trails. These were not the emaciated, desperate bears of climate change documentaries; these were massive, healthy predators, lords of the ice, curious and utterly unafraid.

If this happened during school hours, you, as a student, would only become aware of it when you glanced out the window and noticed something strange: local police vehicles arriving, officers moving with calm but urgent purpose. Then you would see them chaining the doors of the school shut from the outside. This was not to keep students in, in the usual sense of lockdown drills. This was a dual-purpose measure: to prevent a polar bear from being able to easily push through the doors and enter the building, and to keep us students safely inside, away from the potential danger roaming the streets. We'd press our faces to the windows, a strange mix of fear and fascination coursing through us, watching the great white shape amble past, its head swinging slowly, indifferent to the human settlement it had wandered into. The bear owned this land. We were merely borrowing it.

Throughout my mid and late teens, I would become deeply involved in hunting-not for polar bear, as the Inupiat were the only ones permitted by law to hunt them, a right reserved through generations of tradition and necessity, but for caribou and a large variety of other animals I had never had the opportunity to hunt in the past. This was not recreation in the sense I'd known in Colorado; this was participation in the rhythm of life that had sustained people here for thousands of years.

My father had a friend—an employee at the hospital he administered-named Randy. Randy was another transplant, a white person who had originated from the lower forty-eight, but he had married a native woman from the area. That marriage gave him rights and access-such as ownership of a hunting cabin up the Noatak River-that most white people would never have. My parents, recognizing the value of this connection, entrusted Randy to take me on hunting trips routinely throughout the winter months.

Sometimes these hunting trips would have us away from the community for a couple of days at a time. We would load our snowmobiles with supplies and head north, crossing the frozen

Kotzebue Sound, following the course of the Noatak River as it wound through the white expanse. Our destination was a small cabin approximately thirty miles upriver, a simple structure of wood and insulation, heated by a wood stove, surrounded by nothing but tundra and sky. Through these hunting trips, primarily for caribou, I would learn and understand the living habits of other animals-how to detect their presence, how to read the tracks in the snow, how to understand the wind and its relationship to prey. I would also learn, through Randy's patient instruction, the absolute, non-negotiable importance of making sure your snowmobile was in perfect operational condition before making these trips. Out there, thirty miles from the nearest settlement, with darkness and cold as your only companions, a breakdown was not an inconvenience. It was a matter of life and death.

This lesson was reinforced through another part of learning the Inupiat culture within the school system: understanding what you should do if your snowmobile ever broke down between communities, far from any help. The closest community to Kotzebue was approximately forty-five miles away-a small village called Noorvik, home to less than a thousand people, invisible across the frozen expanse. The teachers and elders drilled into us the protocols: stay with your machine, it's your shelter and your signal. Conserve your fuel. Use your emergency supplies. And know that the land, while harsh, also provides.

Randy himself was a man of very short stature. Even at my own age of sixteen, I towered over him by at least a foot. But his small frame belied a deep well of knowledge and resilience. He was another white individual who had found his place in this world, and through his marriage, he had gained a foothold in a culture that was not his by birth. He treated me not as a kid to be babysat, but as a partner, a student, someone worth teaching.

One of the most profound differences I came to understand was the concept of land and property. As opposed to the fenced divisions you would find in the lower forty-eight states, properties in northern Alaska were not marked by boundaries. There were no "No Trespassing" signs nailed to trees-because there were no trees. You were free to roam across the vast expanse, as long as you didn't cause harm or damage to other people's property or disturb their hunting or trapping lines. And it wasn't unusual-in fact, it was expected-that in an emergency, you could temporarily take shelter in someone's abandoned cabin to protect yourself from the weather and Mother Nature's fury. These cabins, stocked with dry wood and basic supplies, were an unspoken network of survival, a testament to the understanding that out here, your neighbor might be the one who saves your life.

During the summertime, when the sun circled endlessly and the tundra erupted in a brief, brilliant explosion of green and wildflowers, I did a lot of camping on my own, without Randy. I had obtained cabin tents, typically made of heavy, breathable canvas that could withstand the wind and rain. I would pack my snowmobile-now converted to wheels for the summer ground—and head out into the tundra, setting up camp in areas within ten to fifteen miles of Kotzebue. I would typically bring one or both of my younger siblings, Meaghan or Pieter, along with a couple of the friends I had accumulated since moving to the community. We would be gone for three to five days, living off the land as much as possible, exploring, fishing, simply existing in that vast, open world. And my parents trusted me with this. They trusted me, at sixteen, to take their younger children out onto the tundra, to keep them safe, to bring them home. That trust was a gift, a recognition that I had become someone capable of surviving in this place. It was a feeling I had rarely known before.

My personal friends in Kotzebue consisted of only about a half a dozen people that I clung to throughout my time in Alaska. In a community of roughly three thousand, everyone knew everyone, but these were the ones who became my tribe, my anchors in this strange new world.

My best friend was Iriuruq-also known as Kim, or Iri for short, a shortening of his beautiful Inupiaq name. He was half Inupiat and half white, a blend of two worlds that gave him a unique perspective. His father, Kim Sr., was originally from Florida-a place so utterly unlike Kotzebue that I couldn't imagine the culture shock he must have experienced-and he served as the commander of our state police post there in Kotzebue. His mother, Vernetta, was Inupiat and worked at the local museum and tourist company, a keeper and sharer of the region's rich cultural heritage.

My second best friend was named Tyson, originally from Oregon. His father worked at the local airport, a lifeline to the outside world, and his mother worked for our local television station, bringing news and entertainment to our isolated community. Then there was my friend Jeremy, whose family had come from Texas. Jeremy was originally friends with Iriuruq, but had attached himself to me when I met Iri, forming a trio that would become inseparable. And then I had a couple of other various friends who filled out the circle: Tommy, Jeff, and Clay, each bringing their own energy and stories to our group.

My first friend of the bunch, the one who would become closest to my heart, was Iriuruq himself. And at first, it wasn't a friendly situation at all. It's kind of weird, thinking about it now from the distance of decades, but it seemed to be a pattern throughout my past: some of the best friends I ever had did not start out friendly. There was always some friction, some misunderstanding, some clash that preceded the bond. Looking back, I wonder if that was because we were all, in our own ways, outsiders trying to find our place—and sometimes the only way to test a connection was to push against it first.

But before I can tell you how Iri and I became friends, I have to explain the context of that first encounter. It requires understanding a very specific time of year in the Arctic.

During the winter months, the snow does not go away. It accumulates, drifts, reshapes the world into a white, rolling landscape. But eventually, spring arrives-if you can call it that. Kotzebue was no exception to the seasonal cycle, but our version of spring was unlike anything I'd experienced in Michigan or Colorado. The issue is this: even during the summer months, when there is no snow, the average temperature hovers between 60 and 70 degrees Fahrenheit. And beneath the surface, permafrost-permanently frozen ground- resides only about a foot deep into the soil or tundra. This frozen layer acts like a solid pan, impermeable to water.

So when all the snow melts-and in the Arctic, it melts fast, the sun working 24 hours a day—the water has nowhere to go. It cannot escape into the ground because of that permafrost barrier. And therefore, the roads throughout the community suddenly transform. They become rivers, small lakes, impassable channels of silty, muddy water. Throughout the entire couple of months of summer, gas-powered generators hum constantly, hooked to pumps that work day and night to push water off the roads, out of your backyard, and into the nearby ocean. Rather than calling it springtime, we called it mud season. For obvious reasons.

There was one particular spring day, my first real experience of this phenomenon, when most of the dirt roads throughout the community had become these rivers of muck. A few stubborn snow banks still remained in shaded spots, but the transformation was well underway. For a teenager like myself at the time, this was not an inconvenience. It was an opportunity. The snowmobiles that had carried us through the winter were now parked, replaced by ATVs-Honda FourTraxes and similar machines-that could navigate the mud and slop. My family had one, and I intended to use it to its full potential.

I went out on that Honda FourTrax with one goal in mind: to sling mud in every direction I possibly could. It was fun, dirty, liberating-a drastic, glorious change from the frozen, monochrome season we had just escaped. The machine churned through the brown slurry, rooster tails of mud spraying behind me, coating everything in their path. I felt like a kid unleashed.

During one of these muddy adventures, as I was traveling down one of the submerged roads, I saw ahead of me two individuals standing off to the side. They were on foot, trying to pick their way along the edge of the road, attempting to stay as clean as possible while navigating the mess. Personally, in my teenage mind, I saw this as a prime opportunity. Targets. People to sling mud at. At least to me, in that moment, the idea was hilarious-just a little prank on someone I probably didn't know and would never see again. Harmless fun.

As I approached them, maybe thirty or forty feet away, they finally turned and noticed me on the Honda FourTrax headed in their direction. They stood still and watched as I got closer, probably hoping I'd stay in the center of the road and leave them be. They had no idea what was coming. Just as I caught up to them, I purposely steered into the deepest mud puddle directly in front of them. The explosion of brown, messy, wet mud engulfed them completely. I remember the satisfying splat and their startled screams as they were drenched from head to toe.

I drove off quickly, looking back over my shoulder, and saw them shaking with fury, heard their yells, and watched as middle fingers shot into the air aimed directly at me. For whatever reason-the thrill of it, the sheer rebellion-this was a trigger for me to turn around and give them a second run. They couldn't even get away from that road fast enough. They scrambled, slipping in the mud, trying to escape, but I was on them again in seconds, circling back and hitting another puddle, coating them with another thick, satisfying layer of mud. Their screams this time were pure rage.

I roared off into the distance, laughing uncontrollably, the mud-covered figures shrinking in my rearview mirror, their fists still shaking. I had no idea, in that moment, that one of those furious, mud-soaked boys would become my best friend. That boy was Iriuruq.

The following morning was a typical morning in Kotzebue. The sun, already circling endlessly in the May sky, streamed through our windows at an hour that felt arbitrary-day and night had lost their meaning weeks ago. I went through my usual routine, my mind occupied with the approaching end of the school year. We were in the early weeks of May, and school would typically end toward the end of the month. The countdown was on. I had completely, momentarily forgotten about my mud-stunt from the day before. In the grand scheme of teenage concerns, it had already been filed away as a funny memory, a story to tell, not a pending consequence.

I made my journey from our house, walking the familiar path that took me through the hospital-the only obstacle between our residence and the middle/high school. The hospital was a shortcut and a warm refuge on cold mornings, its corridors smelling of antiseptic and coffee. I emerged from its far side, crossed the short expanse of frozen ground, and walked through one of the end hallway doors into the school.

As usual, I looked down at the floor as I made my way to my locker. This was a habit ingrained since childhood —my balance had never been good, a lingering effect of whatever undiagnosed condition governed my body. Focusing on the floor in front of my feet was always a priority, a way to ensure I didn't accidentally collide with other students or trip over the scattered backpacks and boots that littered the hallways. I moved in my own small bubble of awareness, the world above the floor a secondary concern.

After entering the building, I walked down a path approximately thirty feet and then took a left down another hallway that led to my locker. The fluorescent lights hummed overhead, the usual murmur of student voices filling the space. I was perhaps ten feet from my locker when it happened.

My left shoulder was abruptly, forcefully slammed into by someone else's shoulder. The impact was intentional -I knew that instantly. No accidental brush, no crowded hallway jostle. This was a statement. I stumbled slightly, my balance wavering, and looked up abruptly to see the faces of my attackers, ready to apologize for what I assumed must have been my fault.

The words died in my throat.

Two individuals stared back at me, their faces inches from mine. I didn't recognize their faces immediately- my memory for names and faces had always been spotty, another quirk of my wiring. But somehow, in the back of my mind, something clicked. My eyes dropped to their clothes. And I recognized the mud-covered garments. Particularly, I recognized one of them—the one wearing a distinct black leather coat that had been absolutely caked in brown sludge the day before.

The looks on their faces made my stomach drop. This was it. This was the consequence. Their expressions were hard, unreadable, but the set of their jaws, the directness of their stare-it all screamed that they wanted to fight me right there and then. My heart pounded. I'd been in scraps before, but never in a school hallway, never with this kind of premeditated energy.

But instead of throwing a punch, the one in the leather coat-Iriuruq, though I didn't know his name yet-spoke. He wanted me to go outside with them, behind the school. They wanted to have a cigarette and talk. Break with me. His voice was calm, controlled. This wasn't an ambush; it was an invitation.

I nodded, not trusting my voice. I quickly turned to my locker, spun the combination, dropped my bag inside, and slammed the door shut. Then I turned and followed them out the door, every step feeling like a walk toward my own beating. I was convinced, absolutely convinced, that I was about to get into a fight behind that school, that my muddy prank was about to come due in bruises and blood.

We stepped out into the cool May air, the sun bright and endless, and walked to a spot behind the building where students gathered for surreptitious smoke breaks. The one in the leather coat-Iri-patted his pockets, then looked at his companion with a questioning expression. He didn't have cigarettes on him. He asked his companion for one.

Without thinking, without calculating, I immediately pulled a cigarette from my own pocket and extended it toward him. It was an instinct, a reflex of politeness in a moment of high tension. He looked at me, surprise flickering across his face, and then he took it.

"Thanks," he said. Just that. Simple. Human.

He lit it, took a drag, and then we stood there for a moment in silence, the three of us, the smoke curling up into the endless daylight. Then we talked. Not a fight. Not even an argument. We had a brief conversation about the day before. He didn't yell. He didn't threaten. He just stated, plainly, that what I'd done was a dick move. His companion nodded in agreement. But there was something else in their demeanor-curiosity, maybe. They seemed interested in getting to know me better. And I, standing there with my heart still hammering but beginning to slow, realized I was interested in getting to know them too.

It was not a threatening conversation. But it was clear: they were not happy about the mud incident. And it was equally clear that something else was happening here. A door was opening. We talked for a few more minutes, about school, about where we were from, about nothing at all. And when we finally crushed our cigarettes underfoot and headed back inside, I walked into that school not as their target, but as something else entirely. Someone they might, possibly, call a friend.

All in the mix of that same time period—the muddy beginnings, the tentative friendships, the slow process of finding my place-another dimension of my life was taking shape. Since elementary school in Michigan, I had always been two years older than most of my peers, a gap that never closed, a quiet marker of the different path my education had taken. On the side of school, or outside of school entirely, in addition to my friendship with Iriuruq and Jeremy growing into something real and lasting, I had taken my first deliberate steps into the medical field.

I was just finishing the ninth grade at the age of sixteen. I was about to embark into the tenth grade. My new friends were one grade behind me-Iri and Jeremy, both a year younger in school, though the gap in our ages felt irrelevant in the face of our growing bond. But at this time of my life, a new identity was forming alongside that of student and friend: I was becoming a medical provider.

In Alaska, the lowest medical certification for entering the local EMS service is an ETT license-Emergency Trauma Technician. It was the entry point, the first rung on a ladder that could lead much higher. To achieve this, I began participating in courses at the Chukchi College campus, a satellite of the University of Alaska Fairbanks, or UAF. The campus was modest by lower forty-eight standards, but it held real classrooms, real instructors, real opportunities. My participation there was focused entirely on training in the medical field, and I threw myself into it with an intensity that surprised even me.

It didn't take long before my ETT license evolved into something more substantial: an EMT license. In Alaska, the system is structured into three distinct levels: EMT-1, EMT-2, and EMT-3. Each level brought more responsibility, more knowledge, more capability. Initially, when I first started down this path, my mother-Mary- and my brother Berend also took EMT courses alongside me. It was as if we were becoming the medical family, with my father serving as the administrator of the hospital and the rest of us training to work within the very system he oversaw. There was something fitting about it, something that made our family feel cohesive and purposeful in a way it hadn't always been.

Some of the elective-related classes at Kotzebue High School were replaced with credits I was earning at the local college campus. The administration worked with me, recognizing that my path was different, that the classroom wasn't the only place I was learning. So it became routine: I would leave the high school at some portion of the day, walking across the small village-past the cluster of houses, past the dog teams chained in yards, past the ever-present view of the frozen sound-to the campus on the other side. There, I would participate in the courses required for my EMT certifications. Some of these courses also took place at the local fire and ambulance service, which was, by a stroke of convenience, located directly across the street from our own house. I could literally walk out my front door, cross the road, and step into the world of emergency response.

My medical experiences during this time would bring me into encounters where human life hung in the balance on a regular basis. This was not theoretical training; this was real, raw, immediate. And when you're living in a small community of roughly three thousand people, your patient is rarely a stranger. Often, it was someone you knew-a classmate's parent, a neighbor, an elder you'd seen at the store just yesterday. Sometimes it was someone you only knew of, a face attached to a name you'd heard in passing. But the connection was always there, always personal. This was a field of expertise that constantly pulled emotional strings deep within your mind, a profession that could leave you with what felt like a twisted stomach or persistent cramps long after the call was over. The weight of knowing the person on the stretcher, of seeing their family's faces in the waiting room, of carrying that memory with you-it was a burden that accumulated with every shift.

In addition to the health problems I had dealt with since childhood—the mysterious pains, the fragility, the endless questions without answers-things got to be extremely stressed compared to what most EMTs could even comprehend. Most of my medical issues could not be hidden; my hearing aids, my hairless scalp, my small stature all announced my differences to the world. But some of them remained hidden, known only to me and my body: the constant aches and pains that I felt within my guts, the grinding in my joints as different forms of arthritis had already begun to take root, causing issues in my hips, my spine, my knees. I would respond to calls, lift patients, perform CPR, all while carrying an internal landscape of pain that I had learned to ignore, to push through, to pretend wasn't there. The irony was not lost on me: I was training to heal others while my own body remained a mystery, a collection of symptoms without a name.

There was even one point-a few years further down the road, when I had advanced further in my training and experience-that my face would become plastered on televisions across America. Dr. Bob Arnot, a medical correspondent for Good Morning America, had come to Northern Alaska to interview different medical staff, comparing the real medical field in the Arctic to the popular sitcom Northern Exposure. That show, set in a fictional Alaskan town, had captured America's imagination with its quirky depiction of life in the far north. Dr. Arnot wanted to show the reality behind the fiction.

When this incident occurred-when my face suddenly appeared on every television in America-I was in the emergency room on a Sunday morning with a young patient, approximately six years old, who was having seizures. Prior to this moment, all of the medical staff of our ambulance service and the hospital had been warned that there was a probability Dr. Bob Arnot might show up with cameras in hand. We were briefed on different procedures we needed to follow to protect the identity and well-being of our patients if this were to occur. We were told to be aware, to be cautious, to prioritize patient privacy above all.

The last thing I expected was that it would actually happen-and that I would be the EMT on duty when it did. That I would be standing there, focused entirely on that seizing child, when a camera crew suddenly appeared. That I would become, for a surreal moment, the focal point of national media attention while trying to stabilize a six-year-old's life. I remember the bright lights, the sudden awareness that this was no longer just another Sunday in Kotzebue. I remember the strange disconnect between the urgency of my work and the bizarre circumstance of being watched by millions. And I remember, most of all, that child—that small, vulnerable life in my hands-and the knowledge that nothing else mattered except doing my job right. The cameras could roll. America could watch. But that boy needed me to be present, to be focused, to be his provider in that moment. And I was.

My friendship with Iriuruq, over the next few years, would grow into something I had never anticipated, something that would fundamentally reshape my understanding of myself and of love. Up to that point in my life, I had never really taken in the aspect of personal sexuality. It wasn't something I thought about, something I explored, something I even recognized as a part of who I was. In some ways, still to this day, that remains true-my identity has never fit neatly into the categories the world provides. But that friendship between him and me, born from mud and teenage mischief, progressed into something far deeper. It became love. A love that would never end, even after it could no longer be lived. For the first time in my life, I experienced what it meant to truly love another person-not as a friend, not as a brother, but as someone whose presence in the world made my own existence more bearable, more beautiful, more whole.

Although he was a grade behind me in school, he was in fact older than most of the students in his own class as well. The age gap between us was negligible-we were only about a year and a half apart. But in a small community where everyone knew everyone, where whispers traveled faster than snowmachine tracks, we kept our relationship silent. Behind closed doors, in the privacy of my room or his, away from the eyes of family and friends, we held each other. And through that closed door, our love drew deeper and deeper each day. It was a secret world, a sanctuary built from stolen moments and shared glances, a place where we could simply be ourselves without explanation or apology.

Years later, when I would finally-hesitantly, fearfully- come out of the closet to my mother, she would tell me something that shattered me and healed me in equal measure. She said she had always known about Iriuruq and me. She had seen it in the way we looked at each other, in the ease between us, in the joy that lit my face when he walked into a room. And she approved. She had privately embraced it back then, holding that knowledge close to her heart, just waiting for me to eventually find the courage to come out and admit my private life to her. She loved me, fully and unconditionally, even before I could love myself enough to be honest.

Unfortunately, this conversation would take place several years later. And unfortunately, it would take place after the unexpected death of Iriuruq.

But for me in that moment-in the years when we were both alive, both young, both discovering ourselves together-my life with my best friend flourished. We continued to hunt and camp together, the bond between us deepening with every shared sunrise over the tundra, every fire built against the cold, every silent moment of understanding that needed no words. We went camping often during the summer months, when the sun never set and the world felt endless. And as usual, I would include my younger siblings within those trips-Meaghan and Pieter, entrusted to my care, learning the ways of the land alongside us. I knew that camping outside the community, having the opportunity for my siblings to spread their wings and gain firsthand experiences with mother nature, would be something that would stick with them for memory's sake for the rest of their lives. And I was right. Those memories, I hope, remain with them still-the taste of fresh-caught fish, the warmth of the campfire, the vastness of the sky.

During my friendship with Iriuruq, I grew close to his family as well. They became a second home to me, their acceptance wordless and complete. When I first properly met his father, it turned out to be a face I already knew. Kim Sr. was the commander of our local state police post, a figure of authority I had seen around town but never connected to the boy I loved. At one point, when I earned my first driver's license in Kotzebue-a milestone of independence—it would be Kim himself who administered my road test. There was something surreal about sitting behind the wheel with my boyfriend's father in the passenger seat, clipboard in hand, assessing my every move. He passed me without hesitation, and I like to think he saw more than just my driving skills that day.

Iriuruq had three brothers and a few very young sisters. His younger brothers were Tom, about nine years old, a quiet boy with watchful eyes. Another younger brother named Joe, approximately a year younger than Tom, more boisterous, always underfoot. And then there was an older brother named Nasruk, who was my age but in the eleventh grade at the time-a quiet presence, someone I never got to know as well as I wished. The younger sisters were only toddlers then, bundles of energy and giggles who filled their home with chaotic joy. They became, in a way, like siblings to me as well.

My friendship with Jeremy would remain a strong, steady presence throughout these years. We often spent the night at each other's houses, playing video games, talking about nothing and everything. But even Jeremy, close as he was, never knew about the private relationship between Iriuruq and me. That secret was ours alone, a sacred space we protected fiercely. I also had other friends who filled out my world: Tyson Quinn, Tommy Russell, and Jeff Dau-each one a thread in the tapestry of my Alaskan life.

Tommy Russell, at one point, almost became the focal point of potentially becoming another foster child to my parents while we were in Alaska. Within the community of Kotzebue, it was sickening sometimes-the way alcohol issues and drug issues could leave innocent children and teenagers often abandoned by their parents or grandparents. The effects of substance abuse rippled through families, leaving gaps where care should have been. At one moment, my mom had found out that Tommy had been living with his grandmother. He had no contact with his own parents at all. And then Tommy made a statement, casual and devastating, that he hadn't seen his grandmother in over a week.

Tommy was approximately two years younger than me. He had often spent nights at our house, as friends usually do, crashing on the couch or in my room, part of the rotation of teenage comings and goings. But until Tommy said something, my mom had no clue that we had been sending him home to an empty house, to fend for himself night after night. The realization hit her like a physical blow. She got enraged—not at Tommy, never at Tommy, but at the circumstances, at the adults who had failed him, at the system that allowed such neglect to continue.

My mom decided, then and there, that Tommy would stay with us until we could figure out what was going on with his grandmother. She made space for him without hesitation, adding another plate to the table, another bed to the roster. She even visited the local courthouse to potentially seek custody, to make his place in our family permanent and legal. She was ready to fight for him, to give him the stability and love he deserved.

Eventually, Tommy's alcoholic grandmother materialized. She reappeared, disoriented and defensive, and the situation resolved itself in a way that left Tommy back in her care. But my mother's willingness to step in, to open our home and our hearts, stayed with me. It was the same impulse that had brought me into this family years ago-that fierce, protective love that saw a child in need and refused to look away. In Kotzebue, as in Michigan, my parents continued to be the kind of people who built families out of compassion, who saw the abandoned and said, "Not on my watch."

But as the end of 1991 drew near, a different kind of crisis began to unfold within our own home-one that no amount of compassion could easily fix. My father had begun to experience health issues that would quickly escalate into something far more serious, something directly related to the diabetes he had managed—or failed to manage-for several years.

When we first arrived in Alaska, my father had struggled to get his personal insulin on a timely basis. The logistics of shipping medical supplies to the Arctic were unpredictable at best, and there were gaps, delays, frustrating periods of waiting. By the time his insulin finally did arrive, he had already been without it for so long that he had convinced himself he felt just fine. And so, against every medical recommendation, against my mother's pleading, against all logic and self-preservation, he made a decision that would ultimately cost him everything: he nearly completely abandoned his diabetes treatment. He only took insulin when he felt extremely sick, using it as a rescue medication rather than the daily maintenance it was meant to be.

For a while, his body compensated. It always had. He was a strong man, physically imposing, accustomed to pushing through. But diabetes is relentless. It does not forgive neglect. As a result of this constant refusal to care for himself, he eventually became so sick that his doctor there in Kotzebue sat him down and delivered a verdict that changed everything. The recommendation was stark, urgent, final: he needed to move himself and the rest of our family back to Michigan, to be near our extended family. It was not a suggestion for a better quality of life. It was a warning that he was now at the end of his life as a result of his neglect. Michigan wasn't about returning home; it was about being close to family when the end came.

So it was planned. In January of 1992, my parents, Meaghan, Pieter, and our newly adopted sister Alice- a young girl who had joined our family through the same open-hearted process that had brought me in-all moved back to Frankfort, Michigan. They packed what they could, said their goodbyes, and vanished into the sky on an Alaska Airlines flight, leaving a void in our home that echoed with silence.

Berend and I would lag behind in Kotzebue until I completed the school season. The plan made practical sense-I was deep into my EMT training, into my classes, into the rhythm of a life that was about to be ripped away. But practical sense offered no comfort in the dark hours when I lay in my room, staring at the ceiling, feeling the weight of what was coming.

And then, in May of that year, the inevitable arrived. Berend and I boarded an Alaska Airlines flight, our bags packed with the remnants of our Arctic life, and prepared to leave everything I had learned to love behind. As the plane lifted off the runway, as Kotzebue shrank to a speck against the endless white and blue, I felt something inside me tear. My heart, my mind, my soul were ripping apart at the seams, and I had absolutely no control over it. I pressed my forehead against the cold window, watching the land I had come to call home disappear, and one question consumed me above all others:

How was I going to live without Iriuruq?

The answer, in that moment, was that I didn't know. I couldn't know. All I knew was the ache, the absence, the certainty that a part of me was being left behind on that runway, and I would never get it back. The revolving door had spun one last time, and this time it had taken everything.

Chapter 6

This had clearly not been the first time I had traveled by airliner. By now, I had crisscrossed the continent multiple times, had watched the landscape change beneath me from Arctic white to Midwestern green. But this flight-this particular journey-was perhaps the worst experience I had ever endured in the air. It wasn't the turbulence, though there was plenty of that. It wasn't the length, though the journey stretched interminably. It was what I carried with me.

From my broken heart, still raw and bleeding from leaving Kotzebue, to the physical assault that followed: for the next forty-eight hours, I was consumed by what felt like the most intense headaches I had ever experienced in my life. They weren't ordinary headaches; they were skull-crushing, vision-blurring, soul-sapping waves of pain that seemed to reach all the way down into the pit of my stomach with each bump of turbulence. Every jolt of the aircraft sent a fresh spike through my head, and my stomach churned in sympathetic agony. I sat in my seat, eyes closed, breathing shallow, trying desperately to disappear into myself, to find some quiet corner of my consciousness where the pain and the grief couldn't reach me. Berend sat nearby, saying little, respecting the wall of silence I had built around myself.

And then, eventually, after what felt like an eternity of suffering, the forty-eight hours of flight came to an end. We touched down in Grand Rapids, Michigan-about four hours south of our final destination-and there, waiting at the gate, were my parents. They stood among the crowd of arrivals, their faces a mixture of relief and concern, and for a moment, the sight of them grounded me. I was no longer in the air, no longer suspended between worlds. I was here, in Michigan, in the place I had come from so many years ago.

By the time we reached our destination of Benzie County -the familiar rolling hills, the dense forests, the great expanse of Lake Michigan-most of the headache and stomach ache that had plagued me during the flight had finally dissipated. The physical symptoms, it seemed, had been a manifestation of the transition, a purging of one life to make room for another. But once both of those elements had alleviated, once my body stopped rebelling against the journey, I was left with something far harder to treat: the raw, unrelenting sorrow of leaving Iriuruq behind. The pain in my head had faded. The pain in my heart had not.

Frankfort, Michigan, is a community of approximately 3,500 people year-round, with a tourist season that can swell the population to nearly ten thousand during the peak months of summer. It is a classic Michigan small town-quiet streets, a picturesque harbor, the kind of place where everyone knows everyone and the pace of life slows to a crawl. For the moment, all of us would be staying at my grandparents' house on Elm Street-George and Margaret Waters, whose home had been a touchstone of stability throughout my chaotic childhood.

Much like my memory of Craig, Colorado, my parents' new house-the one they had arranged for us to eventually move into-was directly across the street from Frankfort High School. The street itself was relatively quiet, with the exception of school hours during the academic year. It was the kind of location that promised convenience, normalcy, a fresh start. But the immediate reality was more complicated.

The house on Elm Street, my grandparents' house, was bursting at the seams. My parents, my younger siblings Meaghan and Pieter, our newly adopted sister Alice, my brother Berend, and myself-all crammed into a space designed for two. There were too many people living in that house at the time, too many bodies, too many personalities, too much history contained within those walls. The close quarters bred tension, a low-grade hum of frustration that none of us knew how to address. We were all grieving in our own ways-grieving Alaska, grieving the life we had built there, grieving the people we had left behind. And we were doing it together, in a space too small to contain our collective pain.

I found myself, in those early days, seeking corners. Small spaces where I could be alone with my thoughts, where I could replay memories of Iriuruq like a worn tape, where I could try to figure out how to be here when everything in me still wanted to be there.

I remember it was within the first week or so of being in my grandmother's house on Elm Street that we found ourselves gathered in front of her television, the family sprawled across the living room in various states of attention. Dr. Bob Arnot's segment on Kotzebue-the one we had been warned about, the one that had caught me in the middle of a Sunday morning emergency-had finally started to air publicly. The first day of the program introduced the concept, the setting, the comparison between the fictional Northern Exposure and the real Arctic. But it was the second day that stopped time.

There, on the screen, was my face. Familiar, unmistakable, staring back at me from the glass. I was there with that young patient, the six-year-old having seizures, my focus entirely on the task at hand while cameras rolled and America watched. Seeing myself that way-objectively, from the outside-was surreal. But the reaction of my family was immediate and overwhelming. My grandparents, my parents, my siblings-they were happy for me, excited that my face was on national television. There was a pride in their voices, a sense that this strange, unexpected validation meant something. That I meant something.

Unbeknownst to me, a large portion of Frankfort and the surrounding Benzie County would also be staring at my face that morning. And that fact would become very well known to me within the next few days, as I took a significant step into adult independence: I bought my first actual car. Not a four-wheeler, not a snowmobile, but a real, road-worthy automobile.

That new car was a 1984 LTD Ford station wagon. It was tan in color, the shade of sand or old khaki, and it drove almost as if it were new. Technically speaking, it was eight years old, but its condition was awesome -well-maintained, reliable, a vehicle that promised freedom. I remember the feeling of the keys in my hand, the weight of them, the knowledge that I could go where I wanted, when I wanted. It was a small thing, perhaps, but after years of relying on others for transportation, after the vast distances of Alaska where vehicles were survival tools, this station wagon felt like a declaration: I was here. I was staying. I was building a life.

Also in that short period of time, my parents secured a mortgage on a new house in Frankfort, at 815 Leelanau Avenue. It was a proper family home, a place to put down roots after years of movement and uncertainty. My parents and my younger siblings would soon move into this house, leaving my grandparents' cramped quarters behind. But my older brother Berend and I were ready for something different. We found a two-bedroom apartment in the nearby community of Elberta-a small, quiet town just across the bridge from Frankfort, with its own character and charm. It was our first real taste of independence, a space of our own.

I had quickly gotten a job at a plant in Frankfort called Frankfort Manufacturing, doing work that was honest if not glamorous. My brother Berend found employment at a nearby gas station called Shell, owned by the Schmuckle Oil Company. We were both working, both contributing, both finding our footing in this new-old place. And then, naturally, we both applied at the local Elberta Fire Department. Given our training and experience in Alaska, we were quickly hired. The revolving door, for once, had opened onto something familiar.

Immediately, everyone in the fire department recognized my face from the news broadcast the week prior. The recognition wasn't or judgmental; it was warm, curious, excited. It raised a certain level of interest among the other members of the fire department and EMS service-I was the guy from TV, the one who had been in Alaska, the one who had worked in conditions they could only imagine. My new neighbors even mentioned it one day, as I was heading out to my car: they had also recognized me from television. It was almost as if, within my very short time back in Michigan, a little bit of fame had come with me.

None of that fame was discouraging. On the contrary, it opened doors to a lot of conversation about Northern Alaska. People wanted to know what it was really like. They wanted to hear about the polar bears, the midnight sun, the isolation, the beauty. And in telling them, in sharing those stories, I found myself processing the loss.

As it usually happens anytime you move on to a new life, the people that you bring into your new world—the ones you work alongside, the ones who share your shifts and your stresses-become close friends. The Elberta Fire Department was no exception. Charlie Thompson would become my new fire chief, a steady presence with a calm demeanor and a wealth of experience. Rick Orlic would become my new assistant fire chief, sharp-witted and reliable, someone you wanted beside you on a difficult call. And then there were numerous other members of the department, each one adding their own thread to the fabric of my new life. We trained together, responded together, decompressed together. They became, in a very real sense, a second family.

Beyond the department, I gained some new side friends who filled out my social world: Mike Holtrey, Bobby Southern, and a few others whose names have softened with time but whose faces remain warm in memory. We'd grab coffee after shifts, talk about nothing and everything, find moments of normalcy in between the chaos of emergency response.

Also, now being back in Michigan, I got to become close to much of my family that I hadn't seen in a long time. Aunts, uncles, cousins-faces that had existed mostly in photographs and holiday cards were suddenly present, real, accessible. There was a comfort in that, a sense of roots re-establishing themselves after years of being pulled up and transplanted. Family dinners, casual visits, the simple pleasure of being known by people who had known you since birth-these things grounded me in ways I hadn't expected.

My father's health-the very reason for moving back to Michigan in the first place-was now being actively treated. He traveled regularly to Traverse City, about a half hour north, to the dialysis center, where machines did the work his failing kidneys no longer could. Despite this, he returned to employment at a hospital in Manistee, a nearby community on the Lake Michigan shoreline. He was no longer the administrator, no longer the man in charge, but the work gave him purpose and provided an income that helped with the mortgage payments on their new home on Leelanau Avenue. My mother worked various jobs around the community to help complement my father's income, doing whatever was needed to keep the family afloat. They were fighting, in their way, to maintain the life they had built.

My brother Berend, now living with me in our Elberta apartment, had also purchased his first vehicle. True to form, it wasn't a practical sedan or a sensible station wagon like mine. He found a good deal on a motorcycle- a sleek, two-wheeled machine that represented freedom and risk in equal measure. My brother didn't ever really own a vehicle of any kind prior to this time, and watching him straddle that bike, helmet in hand, there was a pride in his eyes that I recognized. We were both building ourselves, piece by piece, in this new-old place.

Much like in Kotzebue, my work at the fire department and EMS often involved patients that I knew or were familiar with. In a small community, that's simply the way it is. The person in the car wreck might be the guy who waved to you at the gas station yesterday. The cardiac arrest might be the grandmother of a kid you went to school with. The house fire might belong to a family you'd shared a meal with. And as usual, this would sometimes make fire department calls or EMS calls incredibly stressful, because they included victims that you always knew or knew of. There was no anonymity, no distance between the responder and the responded-to. It was all personal, all close to the bone.

But just like anywhere else, you made yourself get used to it. You learned how to bury the pain that comes with that type of employment. Getting my first medical degree in Alaska as a teenager, I had learned way too early how to hide that pain. I had responded to calls in the Arctic where the patient was a friend, a neighbor, someone I'd seen at the store just days before. I had learned to compartmentalize, to separate the professional self from the personal self, to do the job first and feel later.

Now, as I was turning twenty years old, I had learned the process very well. Hiding the hurt had become second nature. I could walk away from a call, my face composed, my voice steady, and then later, alone in my apartment or sitting in my tan station wagon in a deserted parking lot, let the tears come. I could hold it together in front of my colleagues, my family, my friends, and then, in the quiet dark, feel the weight of everything I had witnessed. It was a skill, learned through necessity, and like any skill, it got easier with practice.

But easier didn't mean easier on the soul. It just meant better at pretending.

With the exception of one period-a year spent in Mancelona after finding my biological family and attempting to connect with those roots-I primarily stayed rooted to the Frankfort community. Mostly because of my family's presence. My parents, my siblings, the familiar rhythms of Benzie County-these were anchors in a life that had known too much motion. The Mancelona experiment was brief, a detour rather than a destination.

There would be another move to Mancelona, but this time my friend Michael Holtrey tagged along with me. The relationship between Michael and I had grown together in a way that echoed what I had once shared with Iriuruq. It was different, of course—no two loves are the same- but the depth of connection, the ease of companionship, the sense of being truly seen-these were familiar and precious. After about another year in Mancelona, we would move together up to Drummond Island in Michigan's Upper

Peninsula, a place of rugged beauty and isolation, where we could build a life on our own terms.

But patterns repeat, and the revolving door spun once more. In the early months of 1998, I would move down to Texas, leaving Michael and the Upper Peninsula behind. My destination was a reunion with a woman named Corina, whom I had met years before in Kotzebue when she worked for my father at the hospital. When I had known her in Alaska, our relationship had been brief but consequential: she had become pregnant with my child. I was only fifteen at the time, too young to be a father, too inexperienced to know what that meant. Now, years later, I would recontinue that relationship and get an opportunity to be around my son, Arnofonso. He was now nine years old-a real person, with a name and a face and a history I had missed. The weight of those lost years settled on me as I held him for the first time.

Shortly after my reunion with Arnofonso and his mother, she would once again become pregnant. Nine months later, my daughter Hope was born. Two children, two lives I had helped create, and a sudden, overwhelming sense of responsibility I had never fully experienced before.

But stability, for me, has never been a permanent state. My relationship with Corina would come to an end before I even knew she was pregnant with Hope. The cause was complex and painful. Corina had an older son from a previous relationship-Miguel-who had become deeply involved with gangs and entrenched in a drug habit that poisoned everything around him. His presence brought violence into our home, a constant undercurrent of threat and chaos that I couldn't accept. I couldn't handle the violence of his gang-related issues, and I couldn't handle the ideology of having drugs within my own home-not after everything I had seen in my

EMS career, not after watching what substances did to families in Kotzebue and beyond. And so I left. I walked away from Corina, from Miguel's chaos, from the situation I couldn't fix. I left without even being aware of her current pregnancy. It would be years before I learned that Hope existed.

I left Texas and headed to Colorado. I soon reunited with my former friends in Craig-faces from a previous life, a time before Alaska, before Iriuruq, before so much. It was nice seeing Craig again, the familiar streets, the sand rocks, the memories layered over by years. This time, I would get a job with a construction company that built hydro and nuclear power plants-a vast departure from any profession I had ever had. The work was demanding, technical, entirely different from emergency medicine. But I made a lot of money, and with that money, I purchased a new vehicle: a 1999 Eagle Talon, a little sports car that was good on gas mileage and fast on the open road. It was a symbol, perhaps, of motion, of freedom, of the ability to leave at any moment.

Eventually, I would wind back up in Michigan again. The pattern held. And then, around 2010, I would move down to Florida, seeking warmth, seeking change, seeking something I couldn't name. I lived there for a period of time, building another iteration of myself in another unfamiliar place.

It would be in Florida that my health would take another devastating downturn. At the age of thirty-nine, I had a massive stroke.

The stroke left the entire right side of my body crippled. In an instant, the body that had carried me through Arctic blizzards, through emergency calls, through years of hiding pain—that body betrayed me. I spent approximately six months in physical therapy, fighting to reclaim what I had lost. Through sheer will and the patience of therapists, I regained use of everything except my right arm. Still to this day, at the age of fifty-two, I have no use of my right arm. The muscles of my upper right chest are atrophied, useless. And there is a complete lack of sensation in the muscular tissues underneath my right arm, stretching down into my rib cage-a dead zone where my body no longer communicates with my brain.

The stroke didn't just take my arm. It took my career in emergency medicine, my ability to do the work that had defined me. It took my independence in ways I'm still discovering. But it didn't take my memories.

With the new challenges of my health came more medical testing-endless poking and prodding, specialists scratching their heads at the mystery my body had always been. And it came with a lot of time for me to reflect on my past. Time I hadn't allowed myself before. Time that forced me to sit with everything I had carried.

My father, once riddled with diabetes, had died right after my twenty-first birthday, on Memorial Day of 1994. His decline had been the reason for our return to Michigan, and his death-inevitable as it was-still landed like a physical blow. It prompted my move away from Frankfort, an escape from something that was too hard for me to bear. I couldn't stay in that place, in that house, in that life, with his absence echoing through every room.

Iriuruq committed suicide right around the year 2000. The news reached me like a blade to the chest. The boy I had loved, the man he had become, the light that had made Kotzebue bearable-gone by his own hand. This prompted me to go through a short bend of depression, though "short" doesn't capture the way grief lingers, the way it rewires you. I learned, once again, to hide the hurt. But some hurts are too deep to hide completely.

My friend Mike Holtrey-the one who had moved with me to Mancelona, the one whose friendship had echoed Iriuruq's in its depth-passed away from heart-related issues. A stent that should have been easy for the hospital to replace ended up being the death of Mike. Another loss. Another name added to the list of people I loved who were no longer here.

My mother Mary, my brother Berend, my sister Earlene -they all died of different elements. Different causes, different times, same result. The family that had taken me in, that had loved me through my silences and struggles, that had given me a name and a place-they were slowly, inexorably leaving. The revolving door wasn't spinning anymore. It was just emptying out.

My little brother Pieter, the red-haired baby born with respiratory issues in 1982, grew up and had four children of his own: Chance, Shane, Clover, and Reno- two adopted, two biological. His older two kids are now passed away as a result of drug-related issues. The cycle of loss continued, indifferent to bloodlines or love. Two of Earlene's three children-Joshua and Warren-are now passed away as well. Her surviving son, Jared, lives in Northern Michigan, carrying his own memories of a family marked by tragedy.

In 2020, I had a second stroke. Since that time, I've been having seizures-unpredictable, terrifying electrical storms in my brain. But at least this stroke didn't take away any more of my body from me. I'm still here. Still fighting. Still remembering.

About six years ago, I learned about my daughter Hope. This news would come to me at a profoundly traumatic moment, when my son, Arnofonso, went to local authorities in Texas to search for me. I would quickly find out, in that surreal and heart-stopping conversation, that I had a daughter-a child I had never known existed-and that my son had been taking care of her.

I would find out the full horror of what had happened. Corina's older son, Miguel-the one whose gang involvement and drug issues had driven me away- had at one point murdered his own mother. He did it in front of my children. Arnofonso and Hope sat in their car and watched as Miguel took their mother's life. At the time of this incident, Arnofonso was fifteen and my daughter was five. Two children, forced to witness the unspeakable.

I would learn nothing about any of this until ten years after the matter, when Michigan State Police knocked on my door looking for me. They informed me that my son was in desperate search for his father. The state police gave me contact information, and I immediately reached out. That phone call-that first voice contact with my son after decades of silence—is seared into my memory. The sound of his voice, grown and changed, but still somehow recognizable. The weight of all those lost years compressed into a single conversation.

Since that time, I have come to know my children. My daughter, who was five when she witnessed her mother's murder, is now an adult. And she has a son of her own now-her son's name is Carlitos. I am a grandfather, though I never got to be the father I should have been. The cycle continues, but so does the love.

All these losses. All these people. My father, my mother, my brother Berend, my sister Earlene, my friends Iriuruq and Mike, my nephews Joshua and Warren, my brother's children Chance and Shane. And yet, here I am. At fifty-two, with a paralyzed arm and seizures and a body that has always been a mystery, I am still here. I carry them all with me-in my memories, in my heart, in the stories I tell. The revolving door may have taken them away, but it cannot take away what they gave me. Love. Belonging. The knowledge that I was seen, and known, and cherished.

And now, I have Arnofonso. I have Hope. I have Carlitos. The door keeps turning, but sometimes, if you're lucky, it brings people back.

Currently, I live full-time in a camper year-round. A choice I made about ten years ago as I fight for my independence-a small rebellion against the limitations my body has placed on me, a declaration that I will not be defined by what I've lost. My camper sits on my late mother's property, in Honor, Michigan-still in Benzie County, still close to the familiar landscapes of my return. The land is quiet here, wooded and peaceful, a stark contrast to the Arctic winds I once knew. My personal camper is my refuge, my sanctuary, my space. It is separate from the home that is now owned by my sister Meaghan, close enough for connection but far enough for solitude. A perfect balance.

I stay in regular contact with my children, normally through video chat, where I get to see my grandson, Carlitos, who is now five years old. Watching him grow through a screen is not the same as being there, but it is something. It is connection. It is love traveling across invisible wires. We discuss the possibility-the wish- that both Arnofonso and Hope want to either move in with me or find a home together. The dream of finally, after all these years, building a real family under one roof. Both of my kids are constantly worried about my health -the strokes, the seizures, the paralyzed arm-yet they are both financially stable in Texas, with lives and jobs and responsibilities. It's a complicated equation, but the wanting is there. The wanting matters.

They also know that I am not alone here. They know that my best friend, Tyler Hines, and his family in Traverse City help me out a lot with basic tasks-the kind of help that independence sometimes requires, the kind of friendship that asks for nothing in return. And another friend, Lance Kingslien, and his wife April, help when they can as well. These are the people who have become my local lifelines, my chosen family in this chapter of my life.

Personally, I am working full-time for an oil and propane company called Blarney Castle-specifically at the EZ Mart in Frankfort. The irony is not lost on me: after years as an EMT, after saving lives and witnessing death, after a stroke that ended that career, I now work at a gas station. But EZ Mart has become like family for me as well. Its manager, Jill Osborne, has created something rare: she has made a gas station into a family-like atmosphere that is genuinely inviting and relaxing. The customers, the coworkers, the daily rhythm-it is a community. It is a place where I am known, where I belong, where my limitations are accommodated without comment. It is, in its own way, a kind of healing.

In addition to my employment for Blarney Castle, I am also a book author. I write about many topics, but the act itself serves as a therapeutic experience as I've suffered many losses and many health issues. Writing is how I process. How I remember. How I make sense of a life that has never quite made sense. The words on the page are my legacy, my testimony, my proof that I was here, that I loved, that I lost, that I kept going.

The camper is small, but it is mine. The work is humble, but it is honest. The connections-to my children, my grandson, my friends, my EZ Mart family-are real. The losses remain, carved into me like the permafrost that never truly thaws. But so does the love. So does the memory of Iriuruq, of my parents, of Earlene, of all the beautiful people who passed through the revolving door of my life.

I am fifty-two years old. I have lived in more places than I can count. I have loved and lost and loved again. I have been a son, a brother, a friend, an EMT, a father, a grandfather, an author. My body is broken in ways that cannot be fixed. But my spirit—that stubborn, persistent thing-keeps going. Keeps writing. Keeps loving.

The camper door opens onto the Michigan woods. The video chat chimes with a call from Texas. And somewhere, in the space between memory and hope, I am still that boy on the porch, watching a goat run past, not knowing that this strange, beautiful, heartbreaking life was just beginning.

I look back now over fifty-two years, and the distance astonishes me. Not the miles-though there have been plenty of those, from rural Michigan to the Rocky Mountains, from Colorado to the edge of the Arctic Circle and back again—but the distance between who I was and who I have become. The boy on that porch in Charlevoix could never have imagined the man sitting in this camper, typing these words. And yet, in some ways, I am still him. Still watching. Still waiting. Still trying to make sense of a world that has never quite fit the way it seems to fit for everyone else.

I think about the Roeters family, about the day they first fostered me in that small northern Michigan town. I was so young then-too young to understand what foster care meant, too young to grasp that I had been plucked from one life and planted in another. All I knew was that there were new faces, new voices, new rules to learn. The Roeters house sat somewhere along the winding roads near Lake Charlevoix, and I remember the way the light fell through the trees in that particular way it does only in northern Michigan-golden and soft, like the whole world was being filtered through honey. I remember the sounds: screen doors slapping shut, the distant hum of a lawnmower, the clatter of dishes from the kitchen where someone was always cooking.

I did not know then that this family would become my family. That what began as a temporary placement would stretch into months, then years, then a lifetime. When they adopted me at nine years old, I became a Roeter in name and in spirit. I gained siblings-older ones who had already learned the rhythms of this household, younger ones who would never know a time before me. I gained parents who signed papers and made promises, who stood before a judge and swore to love me as their own. And they did. God, how they did.

But love, I have learned, does not protect you from watching. From witnessing.

I think about the pain my family saw me endure through those growing-up years. The medical mysteries that no doctor could quite solve. The hair that never grew like other boys' hair. The hearing that faded in ways that came and went, unpredictable as northern weather. The aches that settled into my bones and joints like uninvited guests who refused to leave. My parents sat beside me in so many hospital rooms-white walls, fluorescent lights, the smell of antiseptic and fear. They held my hand during tests. They translated doctor-speak into something a child could understand. They drove me home afterward, and I would catch them looking at me in the rearview mirror with something in their eyes that I could not name back then.

Now I can name it. It was agony.

The particular agony of loving someone you cannot fix. Of sitting helpless while your child suffers, while your mind races through every possible solution and comes up empty. I know this now because I have lived long enough to understand what they must have felt. I have sat beside my own children in moments of pain. I have felt that same clawing helplessness, that same desperate wish to trade places, to absorb the hurt into my own body if only it would spare theirs.

I wish, every single day, that my parents were still alive. Not for anything dramatic-not for some grand reconciliation or final conversation. Just to tell them. Just to sit across from them in some kitchen somewhere, maybe over coffee, maybe in silence, and let them know that I understood. That I see now what I could not see then. That their love was not wasted. That every hospital wait, every sleepless night, every worried glance in that rearview mirror—l carry all of it with me. It made me who I am.

But they are gone. And I am here.

It is confusing sometimes, looking at how life is today. I was once one of the middle children-sandwiched between older siblings who knew more than I did and younger ones who looked up to me. I existed within a structure, a family tree with deep roots and spreading branches. There was order to things. There was a natural progression: parents above, children below, everyone in their place. I took it for granted, as children do. I assumed it would always be that way.

Now I am the oldest surviving individual in my immediate family. The branches have thinned. The tree has been pruned by time and tragedy, and I am left here, looking back at the shape of what once was. I know that somewhere-hopefully not in the near future, but inevitably-it will be my turn to join them. To find out what comes next, if anything. To see my parents again, if such things are possible.

With this thought comes another, harder one. I think about my young nephews who have already passed. Children. Boys with their whole lives ahead of them, cut down before they had a chance to become men. I wonder why. I wonder why my God would take them before me. I am not special. I am not more deserving. If anything, I have had my fifty-two years-fifty-two years of strange and beautiful and heartbreaking life-while they had barely a fraction of that. It makes no sense. It defies the logic I want to impose upon the universe.

And yet. And yet.

I look at the devastation our world is in now. The politics, the constant warfare threatening to spiral into something larger, the hatred that bleeds across every screen every single day. It is enough to make a person want to retreat entirely, to pull up the drawbridge and wait for it all to pass. Some days I do retreat. Some days the camper feels less like a home and more like a fortress, a last stand against everything outside these thin aluminum walls.

But then the door opens onto the Michigan woods. The video chat chimes with a call from Texas-my children, my grandson, proof that life continues. And somewhere, in the space between memory and hope, I am still that boy on the porch. Still watching. Still wondering. Still not knowing what comes next.

That, perhaps, is the only thing that has never changed.

Perhaps the biggest thing in this world that helps keep my mind focused is my employment with Blarney Castle in Frankfort. It's just a gas station-a place where people stop for fuel and snacks, where tires get aired up and directions get asked, where the coffee is hot and the conversation is free. But it's more than that to me. It's a tether, a reason to get up and move when my body would rather stay still. The routine of it—the familiar faces, the predictable rhythms, the simple satisfaction of showing up and doing honest work-holds me together in ways that are hard to explain. When I'm behind that counter, I'm not just a man with a poisoned history and a body that hurts. I'm an employee. I'm useful. I'm part of something.

And then there's Jill Osborne, my manager. Jill has been more than a boss through all of this. She's been steady when my own life has felt anything but. She understands when my health flares up, when the pain rises to levels that make concentration nearly impossible, when I need to sit or step away or simply breathe through it. Not every employer would offer that grace. Not every person would look at someone with my history and see capability instead of liability. Jill does. She sees me. And that matters more than I can put into words. I show up for Blarney Castle, yes-but I also show up because Blarney Castle, through her, shows up for me. A gas station in a small Michigan town, staffed by people who care. It sounds like such a small thing. But small things, I've learned, are often the things that save us.

Then there is this book. This writing. This slow excavation of memory that has become, over time, a kind of salvation. I have been writing pieces of this story for years-journal entries, fragments, lines that came to me in the middle of the night and demanded to be written down before dawn erased them. Only recently did I begin to shape it into something cohesive, something that might one day be held in someone else's hands. The process has been therapeutic in ways I did not expect. To look back at the pain is one thing. To arrange it into sentences, to find the narrative thread that connects one decade to the next, to see the shape of a life rather than just its individual sorrows-that is something else entirely. It is like building a bridge backward, plank by plank, until I can stand on the other side and see where I started.

And I have my siblings. My younger brothers and sisters, still here, still needing their oldest brother. That knowledge sits inside me like a compass needle, always pointing toward responsibility, toward love, toward the simple fact that I am not done yet because they are not done needing me. We lost a handful of nephews and nieces already-children gone too soon, names I carry like stones in my pockets. But others remain. Others still look to me, still call when things get hard, still show up at holidays and funerals and the quiet Tuesday afternoons when family just means being together. I am the oldest surviving member of my immediate family now. That weight is heavy. But it also holds me down when the winds try to lift me away.

The devastating effects of PBB poisoning beat on me every single day. Sometimes it feels like every breath I take is laced with it, like the poison that entered my body before I was born never really left—just settled deeper, found new ways to express itself as the years passed. The hairlessness. The hearing loss. The chronic pain that shifts and mutates, never quite the same from one week to the next, but always present. Always waiting. Some days it is background noise, a dull thrum I can almost ignore. Other days it is everything-the only thing-and I move through the world like a man carrying stones uphill, each step a negotiation with gravity.

But I do not allow myself to cave in.

There have been plenty of times when I could have. Plenty of moments when the pain and the loss and the loneliness converged into something that felt impossible to survive. One time, years ago, I attempted to take my own life. I will not describe it here-some things are too heavy for words-but I will say this: that attempt failed. And I have spent the years since learning to be grateful for that failure. Learning to see it not as a botched ending but as an unexpected beginning. The man I am today would not exist if that younger man had succeeded. And despite everything, despite the pain and the grief and the confusion about why I am still here while others are not, I have come to believe that my existence still matters. That I still have things to do. People to love. Stories to tell.

I live alone in my camper, surrounded by Michigan woods that change with every season. In summer, the green presses close against the windows. In autumn, the colors burn. In winter, the snow hushes everything, and I wake to a world rendered silent and new. It is a small space- bed, kitchen, table, not much else—but it is mine. And I am not entirely alone.

I have Sweettooth.

She is just a house cat, gray and black striped, with eyes that seem to hold more understanding than any animal's should. I named her for her personality, for the way she approaches life with a kind of gentle curiosity, always sniffing, always investigating, always ready to purr if you scratch behind her ears just right. But the name has taken on deeper meaning over time. She is sweet. And she is, in her quiet feline way, a kind of tooth-something that holds on and does not let go.

It almost feels sometimes like Sweettooth knows every feeling that passes through my mind. She jumps up on my lap at moments when I coincidentally need someone close-when the weight of memory presses down, when the pain spikes, when the loneliness of this camper life becomes too loud to ignore. She lays down next to me each night, a warm presence in the dark, and her nightly ritual-the circling, the kneading, the process of needing out her side of the bed just so before she finally settles -is comforting enough to put me to sleep some nights. The rhythm of it. The predictability. In a life where so much has been unpredictable, where health and loss and circumstance have shifted beneath me like sand, Sweettooth's nightly routine is a constant. She will circle. She will knead. She will claim her territory. And then she will sleep, and I will sleep beside her, and the world will hold still for a few hours.

Sometimes I think Sweettooth knows that her comfort means something. That she is not just a cat doing cat things, but a presence, a companion, a small furry guardian against the dark. In return, I give her what I know are her favorite meals-breakfast and dinner each day, timed like clockwork because she has taught me that clockwork matters to her. I let her go out into the wooded area around my camper for fresh air as often as she likes, as long as it's daylight. The woods are beautiful, but they are also wild. Predators move through them-coyotes, owls, things with teeth and talons. So Sweettooth explores while the sun is high, and when evening comes, she comes inside. She has learned this rhythm as surely as I have learned hers.

Beyond Sweettooth, beyond the job and the writing and the siblings who need me, I find comfort in watching good family videos. Movies that remind me of simpler times, of laughter shared around a television set, of the way my parents would settle in after dinner to watch something together. These stories help me escape some of the stresses that I think about each day. They take my mind off my own health, which often hurts so much that I need constant distraction. A good film is like a doorway into another world-a world where problems resolve in two hours, where love conquers all, where the credits roll and you know everything turned out okay.

Real life does not offer credits. Real life keeps going, keeps demanding, keeps testing. But real life also offers this: a camper in the woods, a cat on the lap, a job at a gas station with a manager who cares, a book slowly taking shape, siblings who still need their oldest brother. Real life offers the awareness that I am still here, still breathing, still fighting.

The PBB beats on me every day. But I am still standing.

Chapter 7

Though my adoptive family brought me up Catholic, I strayed from the Catholic Church as I grew older. I strayed from anything that looked like organized religion, really. It wasn't rebellion for the sake of rebellion-it was something deeper, something that had been forming in me for years as I sat in pews and listened to teachings that seemed to bend and twist under their own weight. The more I listened, the more I noticed contradictions. Things they preached from the pulpit didn't always line up with the words I read in the Bible itself. And that disconnect, once I saw it, I could not unsee it.

I do not say this to condemn. The Catholic Church gave me a foundation, a language for talking about God, a sense that there was something larger than this visible world. My parents believed, and their belief shaped mine in ways I am still discovering. But somewhere along the way, I needed to find my own path to the divine. I needed to strip away the layers of tradition and interpretation and human agenda and ask myself: what do I actually believe? What is true, not just what was I taught?

That question has led me through a lifetime of exploration. Before sitting down to write this book, Bitter Legacy, I published eleven other books. Eleven. That number surprises me sometimes when I stop to count. Topics ranging from the paranormal to vampires to my past medical experience as an EMT. I even wrote lyrics for several songs that are also published. On the surface, these projects might seem disconnected—a strange mix of genres and interests that don't obviously belong together. But they share a common thread. Through each one of these books, through different characters and settings and plots, I expressed my own personal emotions. I poured my feelings about situations I had lived through into voices that were not my own. I explored interests that I believe should never be ignored, no matter how unconventional they might seem to others.

Writing has always been my way of processing. Of taking the chaos inside and giving it shape. Of saying the things I could not say aloud to anyone who knew me. In my paranormal books, I explored the boundaries between worlds-a theme that resonates deeply with someone who has spent a lifetime feeling like he exists in the margins. In my vampire stories, I wrote about beings who carry something in their blood that sets them apart, that makes them both powerful and cursed. I did not realize until years later that I was writing about myself. About the PBB coursing through my own veins, the poison that entered me before birth and never left. About the isolation of being fundamentally different from everyone around you.

And in my EMT writing, I processed the things I witnessed. The emergencies I responded to in Kotzebue, the lives that hung in the balance, the moments when training took over and I became something other than myself-something capable and focused and necessary. That work taught me about the fragility of life in ways that classroom learning never could. It also taught me about presence. About showing up for people in their worst moments and simply being there, doing what could be done, offering what could be offered.

But above everything-above the writing and the work, above the pain and the loss, above the questions that still have no answers-I believe something. Something that has held me together when everything else fell apart.

I believe that through my past mistakes, whether they were criminal, unintended, or simply the errors of a man trying to find his way, there is one person who walked this earth and forgave everyone who believed in him. Not just the people who deserved it—if such people even exist. Not just the ones who got their lives together first, who cleaned themselves up, who proved they were worthy. Everyone. The thief on the cross beside him. The woman at the well. Peter, who denied knowing him three times and then became the rock upon which something was built. Me. You. Anyone who turns toward him and says, I need you.

I believe that everyone on planet Earth has the option of salvation. Not because we are good-we are not, any of us, not consistently, not deeply-but because grace is not about what we deserve. It is about what we are offered. Freely. Without condition. Without fine print. And I know, through that one man, that one day all my pain will be gone. The poisons that are stored in my fat cells for life -the PBB that entered my body before I drew my first breath, that has shaped every day of my existence since —will no longer cause my life terror. The hairlessness, the hearing loss, the chronic pain that shifts and mutates but never leaves-all of it will end. Not because I will finally find the right doctor or the right treatment or the right combination of medications. But because I will be made new.

Jesus Christ has offered himself freely to anybody and everybody that accepts him. That is the core of it. That is the truth that has survived every doubt, every dark night, every moment when I questioned whether God could possibly be paying attention to someone like me. He offered himself. Not as a reward for the righteous, but as a gift to the broken. And I am broken. I have always been broken. But I am also, because of him, being made whole.

There are many parts of the Bible that are easily misunderstood. Even the Ten Commandments are often misunderstood. Most people look at the Ten Commandments as a list of ten rules that you must follow in order to make it into heaven. Do this, don't do that, check the boxes, earn your way. But that was never the purpose. If the Ten Commandments were specific laws that had to be perfectly kept, it would be literally impossible for any human being to make it into heaven. Not difficult. Not unlikely. Impossible. Because no one- not the most devout priest, not the most faithful believer, not the person who has tried harder than anyone-has ever gone a single day without falling short in some way.

The Ten Commandments are not a checklist. They are a mirror.

When you look into that mirror, you should see what is wrong. You should see the ways you have failed, the places where you fall short, the distance between who you are and who you were created to be. Romans 3:20 says, "Through the law you become conscious of sin." That means the Ten Commandments were not designed to make us feel perfect. They were never meant to be a scorecard we could proudly present at the gates. They were meant for us to understand that we are not perfect. To drive us to our knees. To show us our need for something-someone-beyond ourselves.

That is what Jesus offers. Not a way to earn salvation, but a way to receive it. Not a ladder to climb, but a hand reaching down.

I have spent my life in a body that fails me. In a world that often makes no sense. In a story that has included more loss than any one person should have to carry. But I have also spent my life being pursued by grace. By a love that will not let me go. By the certainty that this is not the end.

The poison will not win. Death will not win. Despair will not win.

Jesus already did that.

I cannot tell you how many times I have woken up in my life feeling overwhelmed. The number would be impossible to count-thousands of mornings, probably, stretching back to childhood, when I first began to understand that my body would never work the way other bodies worked. Some days the overwhelm hits before I even open my eyes. It's there, waiting for me, a weight on my chest that has nothing to do with physics and everything to do with the simple exhaustion of living inside this skin. Other days it builds slowly, gathering momentum as the hours pass, until by afternoon I am carrying something too heavy for any one person to bear.

But through my faith, I have learned something that has changed everything. I have learned that God wants broken men.

Think about that. Not strong men. Not men who have it all together, who never doubt, who never fall, who never cry out in the darkness. Broken men. Men who have been shattered by life and are honest enough to admit it. Men who cannot pretend anymore. The Lord cannot use people who are strong in their own strength, because people who are strong in their own strength have no need of him. They rely on themselves. They trust their own abilities. They do not reach for anything beyond what they can see and touch and control. And in doing so, they miss the entire point.

Believe me, I could not possibly put into a single book how easily I can get overwhelmed. I could fill pages and pages just listing the moments—the hospital rooms, the funeral homes, the nights when pain made sleep impossible, the days when grief sat down beside me and refused to leave. I have been overwhelmed multiple times throughout my life, sometimes so completely that I could not see a way forward. Sometimes everything just feels like too much. The weight of the past. The uncertainty of the future. The present moment, with all its demands and disappointments. And in those times, I want to give up. I have wanted to give up more times than I can count.

Sometimes I feel like I do not have it within my body or within my soul to give the Lord what he wants. I feel empty. Spent. Used up. Like a vessel that has been poured out so many times that there is nothing left inside. And in those moments, I have learned something else: that is exactly where he wants me.

Because when you are broken, you pray more. You have no other choice. When your own strength fails-and it always does, eventually-you turn to something beyond yourself. When you are broken, you listen more. The noise of your own competence fades, and in the silence, you can finally hear. When you are broken, you depend on God more. Not as a theoretical concept, not as a Sunday morning abstraction, but as your daily bread. Your only hope. Your last and first and only resort.

Second Corinthians 12:9 says, "My grace is sufficient for you, my power is made perfect in weakness."

Think about what that means. Weakness is not a disqualification. Weakness is the very thing God uses. Not despite it, but through it. His power is made perfect -complete, whole, fully expressed-in our weakest moments. Which means that when you feel like you cannot go on, you are actually in the perfect position to receive what only he can give.

I have learned this the hard way, as I have learned most things. When you get so stressed out that you break down into tears, that is when you ask God for help. Not after you have pulled yourself together. Not once you have composed yourself enough to pray properly. Right there, in the middle of the mess, with tears streaming down your face and your voice cracking—that is when he is closest. That is when his grace is most sufficient. That is when his power is most perfect.

So even when you feel like you are at your weakest, worst moment in life, God is there waiting for you. Not judging you for falling apart. Not disappointed that you cannot handle it on your own. Waiting. Ready. Sufficient.

I have heard several people tell me that they think the Bible is boring. I understand why they say it. I have felt that way myself, at times, when I have approached it carelessly or distractedly. But the Bible is not boring. The Bible is fighting for your attention—the same attention that you give your cell phone all day long.

Think about what your phone offers. Notifications that buzz and chime, demanding immediate response. Flashy photos designed to catch your eye. Videos that auto-play before you can look away. Alerts for everything from news to weather to what your cousin just ate for lunch. Your phone is engineered to compete for your attention, to hijack your brain chemistry, to keep you scrolling and swiping and tapping for as long as possible. It is loud, bright, and relentless.

The Bible does not compete like that. It does not give you notifications. It does not offer flashy photos. It does not alert you with sounds and vibrations. The Bible is quiet. It sits on your nightstand or your shelf or your desk, and it patiently waits for your attention. It will not beg. It will not barge in. It will not interrupt your scrolling to demand that you put down your phone and pick it up instead. It waits.

If you only open the Bible when you feel like you have extra time-when you have already checked your email and scrolled through social media and watched your shows and done everything else—it will always feel distant. Or boring. Because you are bringing a distracted mind to a book that requires stillness. You are approaching eternal truth the same way you approach a quick news update. It does not work that way.

The Bible is not full of background noise like you expect from your cell phone or device. It is daily bread.

Matthew 4:4 says that "man should not live on bread alone, but on every word that comes from the mouth of God." Bread sustains you for a day. You eat it, and it fuels your body, and then you need more. Daily bread. Not a week's worth stored up. Not a month's supply. Daily. The same is true for the word of God. You cannot read it once and be done. You cannot skim it on Sundays and expect it to carry you through the week. It must be daily. A little each day. A verse, a passage, a moment of stillness in the presence of something eternal.

Your cell phone can fill your mind with ideas or thoughts for minutes. A funny video makes you laugh for thirty seconds. A news article gives you something to think about for an hour. A social media post might stick with you for the rest of the day. But the word of God can fill your soul for life. Not with fleeting stimulation, but with deep, abiding truth. Not with noise, but with meaning. Not with distraction, but with presence.

Yes, maybe the Bible can seem boring sometimes. I will not pretend otherwise. There are genealogies and laws and passages that feel distant from our modern lives. But as the decades grow and technology advances, our brains are constantly seeking more stimulation. Faster. Brighter. Louder. We are training ourselves to need constant input, constant novelty, constant engagement. Against that tide, the Bible requires something different. It requires you to make time. To sit still. To read slowly. To let the words sink in rather than skim past them.

Even if it is just a scripture or passage a day. That is enough. A single verse, held in your mind, carried with you through the hours. A few minutes of stillness before the noise of the day takes over. Daily bread.

I wake up overwhelmed some mornings. I do. But I have learned to take that overwhelm to the one place where it can actually be held. I bring my brokenness to the God who wants broken men. I bring my weakness to the God whose power is made perfect there. I bring my distracted mind to the quiet book that patiently waits for me.

And somehow, daily, I am sustained.

Christianity is not a guide on how to act.

I need to say that clearly, because so many people have it backwards. So many people look at Christianity and see a rulebook. A moral code. A list of behaviors they need to adopt and bad habits they need to break. And if that was all it was, they would be right to be skeptical. They would be right to walk away.

A lot of people think that being a Christian means trying to be a better person. Stop sinning. Be nicer. Follow the rules. Clean up your behavior. Make yourself presentable. And certainly, those things matter. Jesus gave us the perfect model of how to live-he showed us how to love, how to forgive, how to serve, how to sacrifice, how to obey God. His life is the pattern we are called to follow. But if Christianity was just about behavior modification-

just about trying harder and doing better-then we really would not need Jesus.

Think about it. If the goal was simply to be a better person, then Jesus becomes optional. A nice example, maybe. A good teacher. Someone whose teachings we can borrow while we do the real work ourselves. But that is not Christianity. That is self-help with a religious veneer. That is moral improvement dressed up in Sunday clothes.

Here is the problem: if Christianity was just about being a better person, the goal would be to reform yourself enough to earn your way into heaven. But the Bible says something very different. Romans 3:23 says, "For all have sinned and fall short of the glory of God." Not just some of us. Not just the really bad people, the criminals, the ones who have done terrible things. All of us. Every single person who has ever lived, except one. We all fall short. We all miss the mark. We all carry within us something that cannot be fixed by trying harder.

And Romans 6:23 says, "For the wages of sin is death, but the free gift of God is eternal life in Christ Jesus our Lord." Wages are what you earn. What you deserve. What you have worked for and accumulated. The wages of sin—the paycheck we have all earned—is death. Not just physical death, but spiritual separation from the God who made us. That is what we have coming to us. That is what we deserve.

But the free gift of God is eternal life. Notice the contrast. Wages versus gift. Earned versus given. Deserved versus offered. The price of sin is something that we cannot afford to pay. We are bankrupt. We have nothing in our account. And into that bankruptcy steps Jesus.

So what did Jesus do? He lived the perfect life that we as humans could never live. Perfect obedience. Every moment, every thought, every word, every action- flawless. He loved perfectly. He trusted perfectly. He obeyed perfectly. He lived the life we should have lived but could not. And then he paid a price that we could never pay on that cross. He took upon himself the wages that we had earned. He absorbed the death that we deserved.

Second Corinthians 5:21 puts it like this: "For our sake he made him to be sin who knew no sin, so that in him we might become the righteousness of God." This is the great exchange. Jesus, who knew no sin, became sin for us. Not just took our sin upon himself—became it. Identified with it completely. And in return, we become the righteousness of God. Not our own righteousness, which is like filthy rags, but his righteousness. Imputed to us. Credited to our account. Given as a gift.

Christianity is not about trying to climb up to God. It never was. Every religion in the world is about climbing -about reaching upward through good works, through rituals, through sacrifices, through effort. Do this, don't do that, maybe you will be okay. Maybe you will be good enough. Maybe the scales will tip in your favor.

But Christianity is about God coming down to rescue us.

That is the difference. That changes everything. While we were still sinners, while we were still enemies, while we were still completely incapable of reaching him, he reached for us. He climbed down into our mess. He entered our suffering. He took our death. He did for us what we could never do for ourselves.

When you understand that, everything changes.

You do not obey God to earn his love. That would be impossible anyway-his love cannot be earned. It can only be received. You obey because you already have it. Your obedience is not a down payment; it is a response. It is not trying to get something; it is living out of something you have already been given.

And you do not fight sin to prove yourself. You do not wrestle with your weaknesses to show God that you are worthy, that you are serious, that you deserve his attention. You fight sin because you belong to him. Because he has claimed you. Because the one who rescued you is worthy of your whole heart, your whole life, your whole self. The motivation is completely different.

That is not behavior control. That is relationship.

Think about the difference. When you are in a relationship with someone you love, you do things for them not because you have to, but because you want to. Not to earn their affection, but because you already have it. Not to prove yourself worthy, but because they have already declared you worthy by choosing you. That is how it works with God. He does not stand over us with a checklist, grading our performance. He stands with us as a father, loving us unconditionally, inviting us into deeper relationship.

So here is a question worth asking yourself. Not to condemn, but to clarify. Not to judge, but to examine.

Are you acting like a Christian? Or have you trusted Christ as your savior?

Because you can act like a Christian without ever truly knowing him. You can go through the motions. You can follow the rules. You can show up on Sundays and say the right words and avoid the obvious sins. You can be a moral, upstanding, respectable person. And still miss the entire point.

Acting like a Christian is about behavior. Trusting Christ is about relationship. Acting like a Christian is about what you do.

Trusting Christ is about whose you are. Acting like a Christian is about trying to climb up. Trusting Christ is about admitting that you cannot climb, and letting him carry you.

I have spent most of my life broken. I have failed in ways that would make some people gasp. I have made mistakes-criminal mistakes, moral mistakes, simple mistakes of judgment and impulse. I have been overwhelmed more times than I can count. I have wanted to give up. I have tried to give up.

But I have also learned this: Christianity is not about me getting my act together. It never was. It is about Jesus Christ coming down to where I was, picking me up, and carrying me home.

He did not wait for me to clean myself up. He found me in the middle of my mess. He did not demand that I get better first. He met me in my worst moment. He did not offer me a self-improvement plan. He offered me himself.

That is the gospel. That is the good news. Not try harder. Not do better. Not earn your way.

Just receive. Just believe. Just rest in what has already been done.

Christianity is not a guide on how to act. It is an announcement of what has already happened. God came down. Jesus died. Death was defeated. Love won.

And because of that, everything is different. Not just how I act, but who I am. Not just my behavior, but my identity. Not just what I do, but whose I am.

I am his. Broken, overwhelmed, struggling, failing-his. And that makes all the difference.

One of the scariest verses in the Bible isn't about monsters. It isn't about plagues or earthquakes or cosmic disasters. It isn't about judgment day or hellfire or any of the dramatic images that come to mind when we think about frightening scripture. One of the scariest verses in the Bible is about people. Ordinary people. People like you and me.

Jesus said that in the last days, the love of many will grow cold.

Think about that. Not their bank accounts. Not their social standing. Not their comfort or safety or success. Their love. The very thing that should define his followers. The thing he said would identify us-"by this all people will know that you are my disciples, if you have love for one another." That love. Growing cold.

And honestly, we see this happening everywhere.

I see it on the news, in the comment sections, in the way people talk to each other online and in person. I see it in the political divides that have become more important than human connection. I see it in the way suffering is ignored because we have become numb to it-another tragedy, another headline, another scroll past. I see it in marriages ending, friendships fracturing, families barely speaking. I see it in churches where people sit in the same pews week after week but never truly know each other. I see it in myself, if I am honest. In the moments when I cannot muster the energy to care. In the times when my own pain crowds out compassion for others.

When Jesus said this, he was not exaggerating. He was not speaking in metaphors or poetic hyperbole. He was warning us. Telling us what was coming. Not to scare us into paralysis, but to prepare us. To wake us up. He was saying that the world would get so dark, so loud, so stressful, so overwhelming that people's hearts would freeze. Not all at once, but gradually. Slowly. Imperceptibly. Like water turning to ice, degree by degree, until what was once fluid and life-giving becomes solid and still.

Compassion would fade. Kindness would disappear. And love-the thing that should define Christians, the thing that should mark us as different from the world-would grow cold.

Matthew 24:12 says it plainly: "Because lawlessness will increase, the love of many will grow cold."

Here is what makes this so scary. It is not talking about unbelievers. It is talking about us. Believers. People who once cared. People who once forgave. People who once worshiped with abandon. People who once loved God with their whole hearts, until the world wore them down.

The world wears you down. It does. Day after day, year after year, the weight of it accumulates. The bad news. The disappointments. The betrayals. The losses. The constant noise and chaos and conflict. It grinds against you like wind against stone, smoothing away your rough edges, eroding your sharp passions, until one day you realize that you are not the person you used to be. You care less. You forgive slower. You love with more caution, more reservation, more self-protection.

That is cold love.

Cold love looks like caring more about being right than being kind. It looks like winning arguments at the expense of relationships. It looks like scrolling past suffering because you have seen too much of it and you just cannot feel it anymore. It looks like allowing bitterness to take root and grow, watering it with every remembered slight, every unforgiven wound. It looks like losing passion for God because you are distracted-by your phone, your worries, your schedule, your survival. It looks like loving God with your mouth, saying all the right words on Sunday, but not with your actions the rest of the week.

Cold love is subtle. It does not announce itself. It does not arrive with trumpets and banners. It creeps in. It settles slowly. It feels, in the moment, like self-protection. Like wisdom. Like finally being realistic after years of naive optimism. But it is none of those things. It is the heart freezing, degree by degree.

Jesus was not warning us to scare us. He was warning us so that we would stay awake. So that we would pay attention. So that we would notice when the cold begins to creep in and do something about it.

So we have to ask ourselves. Honestly. Regularly. Is our love growing, or is it freezing?

Am I more kind today than I was a year ago? More patient? More forgiving? Or have I become harder, sharper, quicker to judge and slower to understand? Do I still feel the pain of others, or have I built walls to keep it out? Do I still weep over the brokenness of the world, or have I accepted it as normal? Do I still love God with fresh passion, or has my faith become routine, mechanical, going through the motions?

These questions matter because the verse right after that warning says something else. Something hopeful. "But the one who endures to the end will be saved."

Endures. Not escapes. Not avoids. Not coasts through on easy street. Endures. And what does endurance mean in this context? It means a heart that keeps loving. Keeps forgiving. Keeps trusting. Keeps following Jesus even when the world has become dark. Even when it would be easier to freeze. Even when everyone around you is growing cold.

A soft heart in a dark world is a miracle.

Think about that. To remain tender in a world that hardens you. To remain open in a world that teaches you to close. To remain loving in a world that rewards coldness. That cannot be manufactured. That cannot be maintained through sheer willpower or positive thinking. That is a miracle. A supernatural work of God preserving something precious in you despite everything working against it.

And God can give you that miracle.

He can keep your heart warm when everything around you is freezing. He can preserve your compassion when the world would numb you. He can renew your love when it grows tired and worn. He can do what you cannot do for yourself.

So do not let the world freeze your heart cold. Stay close to Jesus. Stay close in his presence. Not just on Sundays. Not just when things fall apart. Daily. Moment by moment. The same way you check your phone constantly, check in with him. The same way you scroll through endless content, scroll through scripture. The same way you seek distraction from your pain, seek his presence instead.

A cold heart is comfortable at first. It feels safe. Protected. Efficient. But a cold heart cannot love. Cannot forgive. Cannot worship. Cannot receive the warmth that God wants to give.

I have felt the freeze in my own life. I have caught myself growing hard, growing distant, growing cold. And I have learned that the only cure is to draw near to the fire. To press into the presence of the one whose love never cools, never fades, never fails.

The world will keep getting darker. Jesus said it would. But he also said that those who endure—those who keep loving-will be saved.

Not because their love is strong enough. But because his love in them is stronger than the cold.

I recently, in my personal life, attempted to go through with a job promotion. I work for a company called Blarney Castle-it's an oil and propane company, essentially just a gas station chain across northern Michigan. Specifically, I work at the EZ Mart in Frankfort, a small town on the shores of Lake Michigan where the tourists flood in during summer and the locals hunker down through winter. It's not glamorous work. It's cleaning up spills and stocking shelves and ringing up customers who just want their coffee and their lottery tickets and to get on with their day. But it's honest work, and it's been a tether for me when little else was.

This promotion would have taken me to a full-time position in a nearby community called Beulah. Same company, different store. Same basic job, different responsibilities. In the process of considering this change, I knew I was stepping into a gas station that was struggling. Not because of customers-Beulah has its own community, its own regulars, its own rhythms. But because of the people currently employed within it. The store had a reputation. People didn't stay there long. New hires would come in, last a shift or two, and then walk out. Sometimes on their first day. Sometimes before their first shift even ended. I knew this going in. I knew the store was broken.

What I did not know was that my deep-seated Christian world was not prepared for the stress I would endure

I say that carefully. Not that my faith was weak. Not that God failed to prepare me. But that I underestimated what I was walking into. I am already a stroke patient. More specifically, I am a two-time stroke patient. My first stroke hit at age thirty-nine in 2013-young for a stroke, but my body has never followed the normal rules. Then my second stroke came in the early spring months of 2020, just as the world was shutting down for reasons none of us understood yet. Since that second stroke, I have been experiencing seizures. They come specifically when my mind and body are physically worn out. When I have pushed too hard, stressed too long, ignored the warning signs that my body sends. The seizures are my body's way of saying, "Stop. You cannot do this. You are not as strong as you think you are."

I had no clue how cold the hearts of people within that store were.

Not customers. Employees. The people I would be working alongside, trying to lead, trying to fix things with. Specifically, two of them. One was the acting manager within the business-the person who had been running things, or not running them, before I arrived. The other was just a cashier, but a cashier who had been employed at that Beulah store for approximately six years. Six years. In a store where people couldn't last a single shift. That should have told me something. That longevity, in that environment, meant something—and not necessarily something good.

My mission, my personal mission, coming into that store was not just to collect a paycheck or advance my career. It was to fix things. To address the issues that had caused so many before me to walk out. To create an environment where people could work without being ground down. To make that store into what I knew Blarney Castle stores could be-places where employees are treated like people, where the work is hard but the atmosphere is not.

I thought I had the strength for it. I thought my experience, my patience, my faith would be enough. I thought I could absorb the coldness and still radiate warmth. I thought I could endure where others had fled.

I endured for a while. I took what I could take. Day after day, shift after shift, walking into an atmosphere so thick with hostility and bitterness that you could feel it the moment you came through the door. The coldness wasn't just in how they talked to each other.

It was in how they didn't talk. In the silences loaded with meaning. In the way cooperation was withheld, information was hoarded, problems were ignored until they became crises. It was death by a thousand cuts, each one small enough to seem unimportant, each one wearing me down a little more.

Until I ended up having another seizure.

My body made the decision my mind would not. shut me down. Forced me to stop. Delivered the message that I had been ignoring: you cannot carry this. This weight is not yours to bear.

After my seizure, I was immediately transferred back to the Frankfort store. The store I knew I was safe in. The store where the air is different-lighter, warmer, easier to breathe. And it is possible that it could be pure coincidence, but the manager in the Frankfort store is a Christian. Her name is Jill Osborne, and she has created something rare. An environment that is very friendly and very family-like. Not in the forced, corporate way where they hang signs about teamwork and expect that to fix everything. But in the real way, where people actually care about each other. Where your struggles are known and met with compassion instead of judgment. Where you are more than just a body filling a shift.

I am proud to say that the Frankfort store and its employees are very much an extension of my family. After everything I have lost-my parents, my siblings to distance and death, my children to geography and circumstance—that matters more than I can express. To walk into a place and be known. To be welcomed. To be safe. That is a gift I do not take for granted.

As I am saying this, it is an example. A perfect example. Of how the world is growing cold.

The Beulah store was cold. Not in temperature, but in spirit. In the hearts of the people who worked there. They had let something freeze inside them-compassion, kindness, the basic human decency that makes work bearable. And that coldness had driven away everyone who tried to enter it. Until it almost killed me too.

The Frankfort store is warm. Because one person, Jill, has fought to keep it warm. Has created an environment where coldness cannot take root. Where people are reminded, simply by showing up, that they matter. That they are seen. That they are part of something.

Jesus said the love of many would grow cold. He was warning us. Not to scare us, but to wake us up. To make us pay attention to the temperature of our own hearts. To notice when we are freezing, and to do something about it before it is too late.

I walked into a cold store thinking I could warm it. I was wrong. I could not. The cold was too deep, too entrenched, too comfortable with itself. It almost took me under.

But I was transferred back to warmth. Back to Jill. Back to Frankfort. Back to the place where love has not grown cold.

And I am still here. Still working. Still writing. Still fighting.

Still warm.

If you are reading this, you now know more about me than most people ever will. That is a strange thing to sit with -the knowledge that somewhere, perhaps far from this camper in the Michigan woods, someone I have never met is carrying my memories. My pain. My love. My faith. You have followed me through foster care and adoption, through the Rocky Mountains and the remote edges of the Alaskan Arctic. You have stood beside me on the tundra outside Kotzebue, felt that first sharp intake of northern air, watched the sun behave in ways that defy what lower forty-eight eyes expect.

You have met Iriuruq. You know the shape of his name, the warmth of his presence, the way first love feels when you are young and far from home and suddenly not alone anymore. And you know how that story ended. You know about the phone call, the silence afterward, the weight of grief that does not fade so much as settle into your bones and become part of your structure. You have sat beside me in countless hospital rooms, fluorescent lights humming overhead, watching doctors come and go with more questions than answers. You have watched my parents age and die-the parents who chose me, who fostered and adopted me, who sat in those hospital rooms and felt the agony of loving someone they could not fix.

You have felt the weight of strokes. Two of them. The first at thirty-nine, young for such things but my body has never followed the rules. The second in early 2020, as the world shut down for reasons none of us fully understood. You have experienced, through these pages, what it means to have your own body turn against you. To wake up and find that something fundamental has changed. To live with seizures that come when you have pushed too hard, when the stress has exceeded what your damaged brain can process.

You have felt the poison. The PBB that entered me before I drew my first breath, that has lived in my fat cells for fifty-two years, that beats on me every single day. The hairlessness. The hearing loss. The chronic pain that shifts and mutates but never leaves. You know now that this is not something that happened to me once. It is something that happens to me constantly, continuously, without relief or reprieve.

And you have seen my faith.

Not a polished faith. Not a perfect faith. Not the kind that has all the answers and never doubts. The real kind. The kind that had to leave the church of my childhood to find something truer. The kind that wrestles with scripture and questions and the silence of God in the darkest moments. The kind that learned, through decades of brokenness, through overwhelming mornings and tear-filled nights, through one failed attempt to end it all and the grace that followed, that God does not want strong people. He cannot use people who are strong in their own strength, because they have no need of him.

He wants people who know they are weak.

He wants people who wake up overwhelmed and have nowhere else to turn. He wants people who break down and cry out because they cannot carry it anymore. He wants people who have finally stopped pretending that they have it together. His power is made perfect in weakness. That is not a comfortable verse. It is not easy to live. But it is true. I know because I have lived it.

I wrote this book because I had to. Not because I wanted attention or sympathy or even understanding. Because the stories were burning inside me. Because the poison that entered my body before I was born deserved a response, and this was mine. Not revenge-revenge requires someone to blame, and blame is too simple for something as complicated as a chemical disaster that poisoned a generation. Not bitterness-bitterness would have frozen my heart long ago, and somehow, miraculously, it is still warm. Not even understanding, entirely. There are questions I will carry to my grave, and perhaps beyond.

But witness. That is what I owed. That is what I could give.

I was here. This happened. This is what I did with it.

And now you are here too. You have borne witness with me. You have carried these pages in your hands and these words in your mind. You have walked through my life, and in doing so, you have made it real in a new way. A story told is a story that continues. A life witnessed is a life that matters.

If you are struggling-and I suspect many who pick up this book are struggling, because the ones who are not rarely seek out stories like mine—I want you to know that I understand. I have been where you are. I am still there, some days. The weight does not magically lift. The pain does not permanently fade. The questions do not all receive answers.

But I have also found this: the world is growing cold. Jesus warned us it would. He said that in the last days, the love of many would grow cold. And we see it, don't we? In the news, in the comments sections, in the way people treat each other when they think no one is watching. In gas stations where hearts have frozen and driven away everyone who tried to enter. In marriages and friendships and families that have slowly iced over until nothing moves anymore.

But you do not have to freeze.

There is warmth available. There is a God who comes down instead of demanding that you climb up. There is a savior who lived the life you could not live and died the death you deserved to die. There is a grace that meets you in your worst moment-right there, in the middle of the mess, with tears streaming down your face and your voice cracking-and says, "My grace is sufficient for you. My power is made perfect in your weakness."

You are not disqualified. You are not too far gone. You are not beyond reach.

The same God who found a broken man in a camper in the Michigan woods is waiting for you. The same love that kept my heart from freezing when everything around me was cold is available to anyone who asks. The same grace that carried me through fifty-two years of poison and pain and loss is sufficient for whatever you are facing.

You do not have to clean yourself up first. You do not have to get your act together. You do not have to pretend you are stronger than you are. Just come as you are. Broken. Overwhelmed. Worn out. Worn down. Wondering if it is even worth it anymore.

Come anyway.

The camper door opens onto the Michigan woods. Sweettooth is scratching at the screen, ready to come back in. Outside, the light falls through the trees in that particular way it does only here-golden and soft, like the whole world is being filtered through honey. The seasons will change again. The tourists will come and go. The gas station in Frankfort will keep selling coffee and lottery tickets, and Jill will keep making it a place where family happens.

The video chat will chime soon with a call from Texas. My children. My grandson. Proof that life continues, that love travels across miles, that connection survives distance.

And somewhere, in the space between memory and hope, I am still that boy on the porch in Charlevoix. Still watching. Still wondering. Still not knowing what comes next.

But I know who holds what comes next. And that, finally, is enough.

The poison beats on me every day. But I am still here. Still warm. Still his.

And now you are part of this story too. You have read it. You have carried it. It belongs to you now, in some small way. Take it with you. Let it remind you that survival is possible. That love can stay warm in a cold world. That weakness is not the end-it is the beginning.

The camper door closes behind me as I step outside to let Sweettooth in. The Michigan woods surround me, familiar and beautiful and full of life. Somewhere, a bird calls. Somewhere, a car passes on the road. Somewhere, the world keeps turning, cold in so many places, but warm here. Warm in this moment. Warm in this heart.

Thank you for reading. Thank you for witnessing. Thank you for being part of the legacy.

It was strange, and beautiful, and heartbreaking.

And it was mine.

And now it is ours.

Don't miss out!

Visit the website below and you can sign up to receive emails whenever Christopher Lee Roeters publishes a new book. There's no charge and no obligation.

https://books2read.com/r/B-A-MATQ-GJKBJ

BOOKS 2 READ

Connecting independent readers to independent writers.

Also by Christopher Lee Roeters

Hybrid

Hybrid

Hybrid: Reckoning

It's In The Blood

It's In The Blood (Book 1)

It's In The Blood (Book 2)

It's In The Blood (Book 3)

It's In The Blood (Book 4)

It's In The Blood (Book 5)

It's In The Blood (Book 6)

Its In The Blood (Book 7)

Standalone

Biblical and Traditional Timeline In One

Angels Among Us

Stories Of A Medic In Northern Alaska

Sleepy Hallow

Music Lyrics
Bitter Legacy

About the Author

Christopher Lee Roeters is a prolific full-time author whose extraordinary life journey shapes the vivid worlds, deep resilience, and profound empathy found across his 15 published books. From the rural towns of Michigan to the freezing, remote edge of Kotzebue, Alaska, Christopher has lived a life defined by survival, service, and an unwavering dedication to truth.

As a former first responder and EMT in Northern Alaska, Christopher experienced the raw, life-or-death realities of the wilderness firsthand—experiences that ground his gripping medical memoirs and fuel the high-stakes action of his science fiction and urban fantasy series. His profound, twenty-year dedication to theological research and biblical studies further enriches his writing, allowing him to seamlessly bridge ancient history, global prophecy, and modern world affairs into definitive reference timelines.

Writing full-time from his home in Michigan while navigating the personal challenges a history of chronic illness, Christopher uses his craft to explore universal themes of found family, brotherhood, equality, and the triumphant power of the human spirit. Whether crafting high-octane cyborg thrillers, deep gothic vampire sagas, or raw autobiographical accounts, his stories serve as a powerful reminder that even in the deepest darkness, light can always be found.

When he isn't expanding his multi-genre literary universe, Christopher composes original music and lyrics tied directly to his books, offering readers an interactive, multi-sensory backstage pass to his worlds.

www.ingramcontent.com/pod-product-compliance
Lightning Source LLC
LaVergne TN
LVHW090404210926
848480LV00002B/439
* 9 7 9 8 2 3 3 8 3 2 3 1 4 *